SUGAR SHOCK

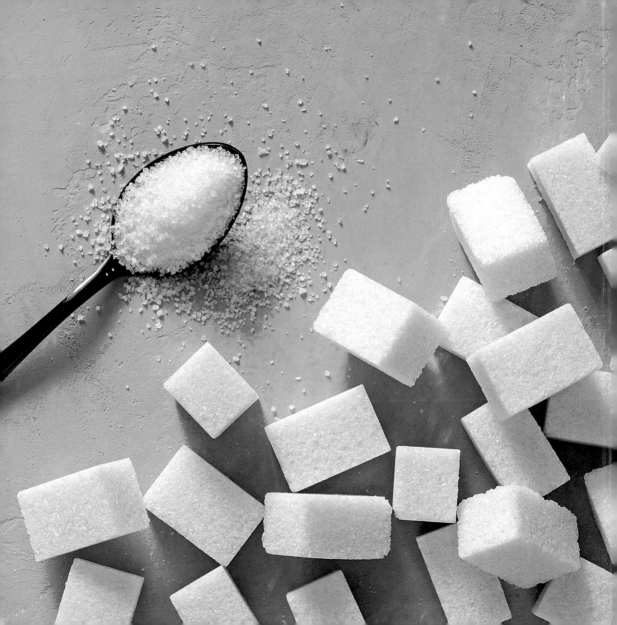

SUGAR SHOCK

THE HIDDEN SUGAR IN YOUR FOOD

100+ HEALTHY SWAPS TO CUT BACK

CAROL PRAGER with
SAMANTHA CASSETTY, MS, RD
FOREWORD BY VALERIE GOLDSTEIN, MS, RD, CDE

HEARST
HOME

CONTENTS

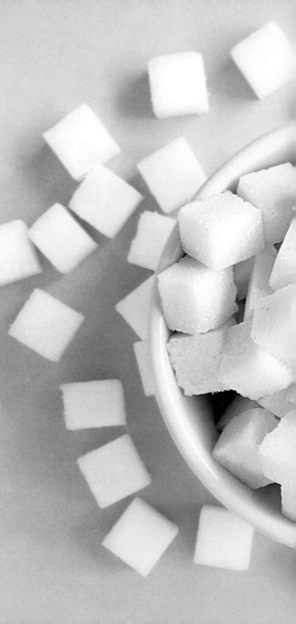

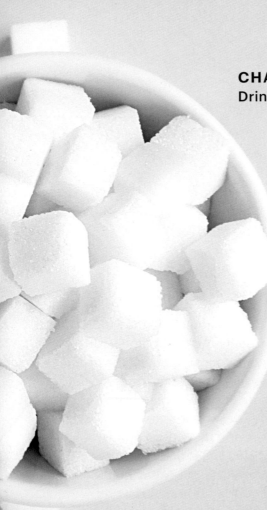

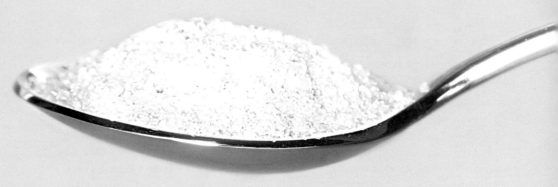

THE ADDICTIVE NATURE OF SUGAR HAS LONG BEEN RECOGNIZED. Today, we are living proof of a syrupy sweet epidemic and its oh-so-sticky hold on us. Americans consume 150 pounds more sugar today than we did 200 years ago. During the 1700s, most Americans ingested only 2–6 pounds of sugar for the entire year. Now we devour 3 pounds of sugar a week! Like Def Leppard's '80s classic, "Pour Some Sugar on Me," the food industry has been doing just that! Pouring sugar into just about all the products they make yet labeling them with words designed to fool you.

We eat super-sized amounts of sugar and most of us don't even know it. *Sugar Shock* exposes this increasingly unhealthy behavior... and will rock your honeyed world.

Working as a registered dietitian and

certified diabetes educator for Long Island Medical Center never prepared me for what I would experience after landing a gig with the famed Dr. Atkins. Although there was very little research then on minimizing sugar and eating more fat, my experiences with countless patients who thrived after making those dietary changes were jaw-dropping. I witnessed firsthand the addiction and the deleterious effects of sugar on patients, and then got to experience how they recaptured wellness, maintained an energy surge, experienced dramatic weight loss, and much, much more.

Regrettably, it is only after Americans have been struggling to battle the diabesity (a form of diabetes associated with being obese) epidemic, and a dangerous rise in blood sugar and metabolic disorders, that researchers finally began investigating sugar's significant role in mental and dental health, cancer, infertility, premature aging, and heart health. Consumers have been blindly overdosing on sugar for decades; it has grown from a luxury treat to the world's most valuable crop and sits at the center of a global health crisis.

Sugar Shock provides a comprehensive understanding of all things sugar. It is an invaluable tool, teaching you sugar's impact on your health, how to read food product labels and providing you with a sugar tracker to track your own sugar intake, and how to find it lurking in your food. It educates you on how to swap sugar for lower sugar alternatives for more than 100 everyday foods. Then, the 21-Day Sugar-Detox Meal Plan (page 83) supplies assistance and support for your transition to optimal eating.

It is no secret we all want to look and feel our best. Cutting out added sugar will help significantly toward this goal. Take ownership of your health and take back your quality of life as we gallantly battle the sugar epidemic together.

—Valerie Goldstein, MS, RD, CDE

IT'S HARD TO THINK OF ANYTHING YOU EAT THAT'S LINKED TO AS MANY HEALTH PROBLEMS AS ADDED SUGAR. The negative effects of excess sugar in your diet extend far beyond weight gain: Too much added sugar can increase your risk for debilitating health problems like type 2 diabetes and heart disease, and in some studies, it has even been shown to reduce life expectancy.

Sugar takes hold of your taste buds and your brain. When you consume too much added sugar, you're primed to want more, and you may become less satisfied by real, naturally sweet whole foods, such as fruit. Sugar also lights up reward circuitry in your brain, making sweet foods seem especially enticing. Studies tell us that being hooked on sugar is similar to being hooked on drugs. This may explain why you crave sweets and why a sugary treat gives you such a thrill.

Hidden sugars in packaged foods make it especially hard to eat well. Even if you skip dessert, your diet is probably riddled with sugar. Americans consume an average of 22 teaspoons (about 88 grams) of sugar per day, far above the American Heart Association's suggested limits. While half of that sugar comes from drinks, like soda, tea, coffee beverages, and sports drinks, the other half comes from food. Sugar is hiding in literally every aisle of the grocery store. Think breads, cereals (even whole-grain versions), yogurt, jerky, plant-based milks, soups, salad dressings, pasta sauces, and more. If your breakfast consists of flavored oatmeal prepared with vanilla almond milk, and an almond milk latte on the side, you've probably maxed out your sugar intake before your morning commute—while eating supposedly healthy fare.

That's all about to change! Right now, you're holding the step-by-step guide to freeing yourself from sugar's unhealthy hold. In *Sugar Shock*, you'll learn the latest science on how your body processes sugar and discover what it does to your body and brain. Then you'll be ready to take action.

Sugar Shock includes a 7-Day Sugar Tracker (page 46) so you can calculate exactly how much added sugar you eat. It'll reveal where sugar is sneaking into your diet (maybe in a coffee drink on your way to work, a soda with lunch, or a jarred pasta sauce at dinner) so you can find a lower-sugar replacement that's just as tasty but doesn't bring the damaging side effects. For *Sugar Shock*, we researched nearly 1,000 foods to find these better-for-you swaps.

We also included a sugar-detox meal plan loaded with satisfying weekday-friendly menu ideas so you won't need to rely on your usual sugar fix.

By cutting excess added sugar from your diet, you may experience benefits such as:

• A slimmer waistline with less belly bloat.
• Improved skin tone and texture, with fewer wrinkles over time.
• Better sleep, which means you'll feel more focused and productive.
• A lower risk for debilitating diseases, so you can feel better as you age.
• More control over your eating habits, so when you're having something sweet, it's a deliberate choice to indulge (instead of a food manufacturer's decision).

We're so pleased to bring you *Sugar Shock*. It's truly your road map to a healthier, more vibrant life.

—Samantha Cassetty, MS, RD

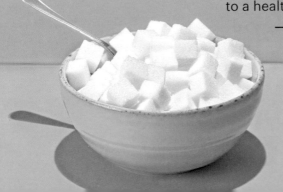

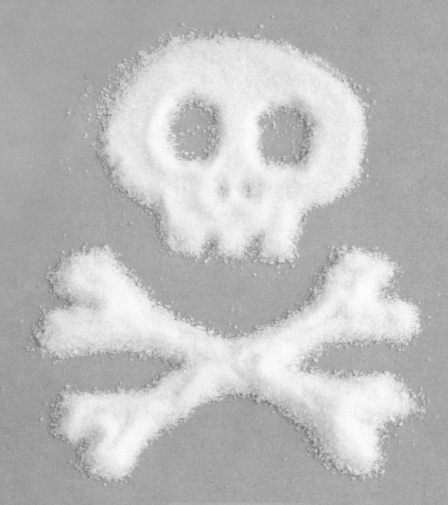

CHAPTER 1

THE DARK SIDE OF
SUGAR

High on Sugar

Here's a shocker: The American Heart Association (AHA) estimates that Americans consume over 110 pounds (or about 22 five-pound bags) of added sugar per year! Break that down to the daily level, and we're way over the recommended limit, downing the equivalent of 22 teaspoons (88 grams) of added sugars a day. The AHA recommends that women should max out at the equivalent of 6 teaspoons (24 grams) of added sugars daily; men should stop at 9 teaspoons (36 grams). If you have any health conditions that are influenced by sugar consumption, it is best to minimize or completely eliminate added sugar.

Naturally occurring sugars—those found in small amounts in fruits, vegetables, and milk—are not the problem. These foods contain important nutrients and are often high in fiber, which slows the absorption of sugar into the bloodstream. The big no-no for your health is the sugar that's added to food and beverages during preparation or processing. Added sugar is almost everywhere in the modern diet, lurking in many unexpected foods we assume are otherwise healthy. That means we're often eating the sweet stuff and don't even know it. The fact is 80 percent of the 600,000 consumer packaged foods in the United States have added sugar, according Robert Lustig, M.D., Professor Emeritus of Pediatrics, Division of Endocrinology at the University of California, San Francisco (UCSF).

Science shows consumption of added sugar in such vast quantities can wreak havoc on our bodies over time. Both the AHA and the Centers for Disease

Control and Prevention (CDC) state that the added sugars in sodas, baked goods, and other processed foods are likely responsible for the increase in calorie consumption and the subsequent rise in obesity among American adults and children over the past few decades. Today, approximately two-thirds of Americans are overweight or obese, according to the Harvard School of Public Health. That's not even the worst part: In addition to its association with obesity, excess sugar consumption has been linked to many more serious health conditions such as food addiction, Alzheimer's disease, cancer, cavities, insulin resistance, high triglycerides, fatty liver, heart disease, and type 2 diabetes.

Enter *Sugar Shock*. This book will give you all the tools you need to help you understand and gain control of the amount of sugar you choose to eat. It'll share the science behind sugar: what it does to you, why your body is wired to crave it, and how to keep track of your intake. Plus, it'll reveal 57 secret identities of added sugar hiding on food labels. The simple 7-Day Sugar Step-Down Plan (page 70) will give you practical ways to start reducing the sugar in your diet. And if you want to go further, the 21-Day Sugar-Detox Meal Plan (page 83) will help you cut out added sugar entirely and includes delicious recipes for breakfast, lunch, dinner, and snacks. Starting in Chapter 6, the Sugar Hall of Shame will reveal which processed foods are the sweetest of the sweet (many of them are made by America's most common brands). But most important, you'll discover more than 100 of the most popular foods with hidden (and not so hidden) sugars and offer lower-sugar swaps, so you can make informed food choices.

We give you the sugar-reducing strategies and solutions for shopping and for every meal. The result? You'll reap total-body benefits as a reward. Now, *that's* sweet.

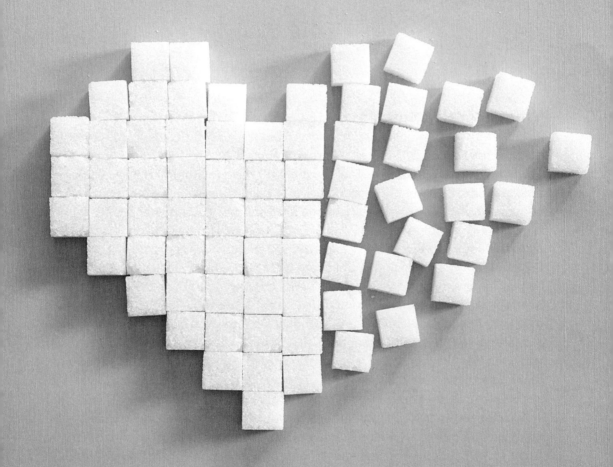

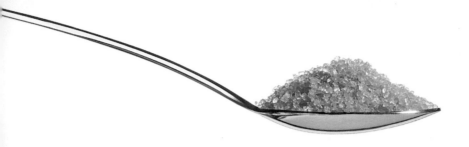

What is Added Sugar?

There are two types of sugars in food: NATURAL SUGAR and ADDED SUGAR. Natural sugar is found in small amounts in fruits, vegetables, and milk, all of which also contain important nutrients. Eating a diet rich in vegetables and fruits as part of an overall healthy diet may reduce risk for heart disease, including heart attack and stroke. Fresh produce is also often high in fiber, which slows the absorption of sugar into the bloodstream, and eating high-fiber fruits and veggies may also reduce the risk for obesity and type 2 diabetes. For the purpose of understanding and limiting your sugar intake, we're not concerned about natural sugar. The big threat to your health is added sugar, which is also known by a host of other names, including high-fructose corn syrup (HFCS) and sucrose (see Fifty Shades of Sugar, page 32). This is the sugar that's added to food during preparation or processing. Your body digests natural and added sugars the same way. However, because food that contains natural sugar often has other nutrients that impact how your body breaks sugar down, there's a big difference.

For example, take strawberry-flavored yogurt. Manufacturers typically add sugar in addition to the fruit to make it more palatable. This added sugar can cause quick fluctuations in your blood sugar levels, which can affect your mood. That sugar kick provides a boost of energy, but it is short-lived. A blood sugar drop will always follow a sugar high, leading to a vicious cycle as your body craves more sugar. These continuous spikes and drops in energy levels can make you tired and irritable.

On the other hand, there's plain yogurt, which contains natural sugar in the form of lactose (see The Science of Sugar, page 17). When you combine plain yogurt (a good source of protein) with fresh strawberries, the whole fruit adds fiber along with natural sugar. Though fruit still adds sugar, this healthier alternative offers essential nutrients that slow down digestion and help you feel full for longer, allowing you to experience less of a blood sugar spike than if you had that sweetened flavored yogurt.

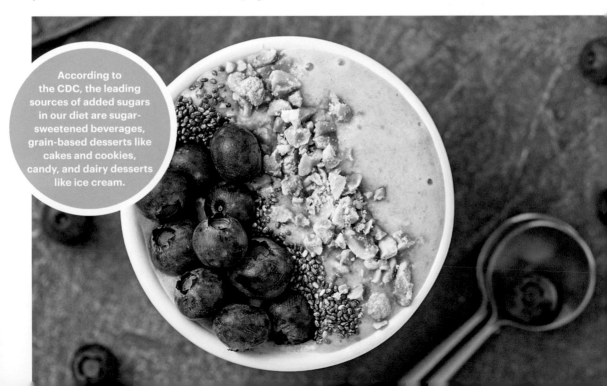

According to the CDC, the leading sources of added sugars in our diet are sugar-sweetened beverages, grain-based desserts like cakes and cookies, candy, and dairy desserts like ice cream.

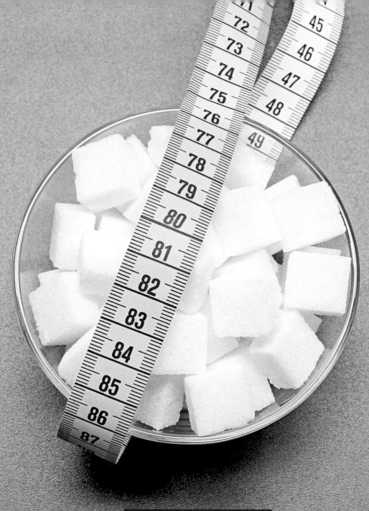

CHAPTER 2

YOUR BODY ON
SUGAR

The Science of Sugar

We're not going to sugarcoat the truth: Your body is wired to crave sweets. That's no surprise if you've tried to cut down on sugar in the past but found it too hard to resist. It doesn't help that you're bombarded with information (and misinformation) about sugar, some of that messaging well-intentioned, but much of it overwhelming and confusing.

Sugar provides empty calories and no real nutrient value so it's not important to our diets: The least amount of added sugar you eat, the better. You consume plenty of sugar from natural foods. Natural sugar appears in the form of **FRUCTOSE** in fruits, **LACTOSE** in dairy products, and **GLUCOSE** in commercially produced starches such bread and pasta, along with plant-based starches such as rice and potatoes.

Our bodies are programmed to crave sugar-rich foods. That was fine in times when sugar was relatively scarce except in its natural forms. But flash forward to today, when sugar-laden processed food is available in affordable abundance: Our normal craving for natural sweetness has morphed into overconsumption of cheap, readily available addictive sugar, which is wreaking havoc on our health. But don't be discouraged. The first step in freeing yourself from sugar's grasp is not to ignore the buzz, but to understand the science behind it. After that, you'll be ready to take The Sweet Tooth Quiz (page 25) to receive important insight into the patterns of your sugar consumption.

SUGAR AND YOUR HORMONES

As part of a healthy diet, very small amounts of sugar trigger a minimal insulin response. As you eat more sugar, it triggers a bigger blood sugar spike in your body and the release of more insulin, a fat-storing hormone. Insulin grabs glucose from your blood and delivers it to your cells to be used as energy. That said, insulin stores one-hundred percent of excess sugar as fat. So when you incorporate sugary treats into the mix? The excess glucose floods your system, giving you a quick but dirty high (a.k.a. a blood sugar spike). Your brain counters by shooting out serotonin, a sleep-regulating hormone, otherwise known as a sugar crash. If you consume excess sugar on a regular basis, over time these sugar highs and lows can seriously stress your system. According to the Harvard School of Public Health, repeated blood sugar spikes create inflammation. If this inflammation becomes chronic, it can trigger a cascade of changes in your body, including the narrowing of the arteries and insulin resistance (when cells in your muscles, body, fat, and liver start resisting or ignoring insulin). This is a medical condition on its own and can be a precursor to diabetes.

SUGAR AND YOUR BLOOD

Studies dating back decades show that eating too much fructose can contribute to unhealthy levels of body fat. Fructose is also stored as fat in the liver. It's not the relatively modest quantities of fructose in fruit that should worry you. High-fructose corn syrup (HFCS), an added sugar, is another matter (See Fifty Shades of Sugar, page 32). HFCS is a common sugar added to processed foods because it's cheap to produce and makes processed foods taste good. Your liver can hold only so much fructose at a time. Just like with any sugar, fill up your tank with HFCS and excess fructose in your system is processed into triglycerides, a type of fat found in your blood. According to a University of Minnesota study, the large amount of HFCS we consume from processed foods and beverages has the most significant (and dangerous) impact on our body fat. By maintaining a healthy weight, most people can keep their triglycerides at acceptable levels. But if you're overweight or gaining weight, triglycerides will accumulate and become a core predictor of heart disease and stroke.

SUGAR AND YOUR WEIGHT

Experts have long known that high sugar intake can lead to obesity. You probably know that too many calories from any source will be stored as fat if not burned. But the lack of nutrients in sugar actually makes it much easier to consume to excess with no physical effects to warn you of potential harm. Foods rich in fiber, fat, and protein all have been associated with increased fullness. Sugar will give you the calories but not the feeling that you've had enough. So when you eat sugary foods, and you think they taste great, remember sugar increases your cravings for more, but lacks essential nutrients, leaving your body less satisfied, making you more likely to indulge again and again.

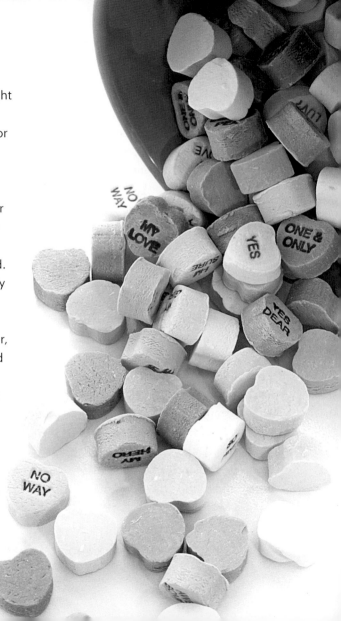

SUGAR AND YOUR BELLY

Insulin also blocks production of leptin, the "hunger hormone" that tells your brain that you're full. Eating sugar raises insulin. The higher your insulin levels, the hungrier you will feel (even if you've just eaten a lot). Now in simulated starvation mode, your brain directs your body to start storing sugar as belly fat.

SUGAR AND YOUR HEART

A *BMJ* Open Heart study revealed that excess sugar may increase the risk for hypertension even more than sodium will. Research also suggests that sugar plays a greater role in heart disease than even saturated fat does. More worrisome, leading an otherwise healthy lifestyle doesn't appear to offset the effect: A *JAMA* Internal Medicine study revealed that the more added sugar people ate, the greater their risk of dying of heart disease— regardless of their physical activity level and weight.

SUGAR AND YOUR BRAIN

While experts have known for years that people who have uncontrolled diabetes (high blood sugar levels) are at greater risk for brain shrinkage and developing dementia, new studies are showing that even those whose blood sugar levels fall short of a diabetes diagnosis, also known as prediabetes, may be vulnerable to these changes. In an Australian study, people with blood sugar levels at the high end of the normal range were more likely to have a loss of brain volume in the hippocampus and amygdala—areas involved in memory and cognition—than were people who had lower normal-range blood sugar levels.

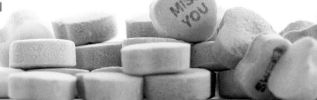

The Sugar Cycle

Loading up on sugar has a powerful effect on the biology of your body—namely, it tricks your brain into wanting more. When you eat sugary foods, the tongue signals to the brain to release the feel-good hormones serotonin and dopamine. These hormones make you crave food and feel pleasure while eating. Here's how it works:

1 Excess sugar enters your bloodstream, causing your pancreas to produce extra insulin.

2 This extra insulin signals your fat cells to stockpile more glucose, fatty acids, and other calorie-rich substances.

3 After stockpiling, too few calories remain in your bloodstream. Your brain, which has very high-energy needs, believes it's now low on fuel.

4 As a result, your hunger level rises quickly. That makes sugar, a speedy source of energy, irresistible, so you crave more of it—even if you've just eaten sugary food.

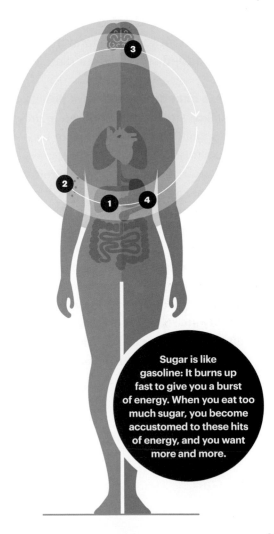

Sugar is like gasoline: It burns up fast to give you a burst of energy. When you eat too much sugar, you become accustomed to these hits of energy, and you want more and more.

Sugars Are Carbs

It's important to understand the role of carbohydrates when talking about added sugar in your diet.

SIMPLE CARBOHYDRATES have basic chemical structures composed of only one sugar (monosaccharides) or two sugars (disaccharides). While some simple carbs occur naturally in fruit (fructose) and milk (lactose), most of the simple carbs in the American diet are added sugar (like sucrose, fructose, and glucose). Simple carbs, such as those found in fruit juice concentrate, regular soda, sports drinks, many baked goods, crackers, pasta, and refined white rice, are quickly utilized for energy by the body, often leading to a fast rise in blood sugar, which can have negative health effects.

COMPLEX CARBOHYDRATES have chemical structures with three or more sugars linked together (known as oligosaccharides and polysaccharides). Many complex-carb foods contain fiber, vitamins, and minerals, so they take longer to digest and have a less immediate impact on blood sugar levels.

THE GLYCEMIC INDEX (GI) (on right) was invented at the University of Toronto as another way of explaining how carb-rich foods affect blood sugar. The GI ranks carbs on a scale of 0 to 100 based on how quickly and how much they raise blood sugar levels after eating. Foods with a high glycemic index, like white bread, are rapidly digested and cause substantial fluctuations in blood sugar. Foods with a lower glycemic index, like whole oats, are digested more slowly, prompting a more gradual rise in blood sugar.

GLYCEMIC INDEX

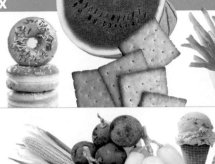
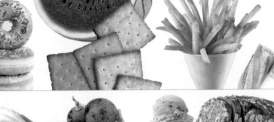

- white bread, donuts, baguette, crackers, waffles
- white rice, mashed potatoes, french fries
- watermelon
- cornflakes

70–100

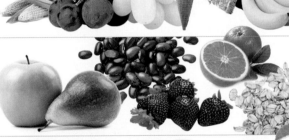

- rye & whole-grain bread
- muesli; corn; couscous; brown rice; spaghetti; popcorn; yams; boiled, roasted & baked potatoes
- ice cream, flavored yogurt
- banana, grapes, kiwi

50–70

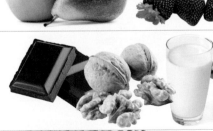

- strawberries, apples, pears, oranges
- soy milk
- unsweetened yogurt
- oatmeal
- beans

30–50

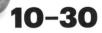

- pearled barley, lentils
- grapefruit, cherries, apricots & plums
- dark (70%) chocolate
- whole milk
- cashews, walnuts

10–30

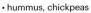
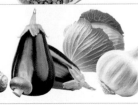

- hummus, chickpeas
- garlic, onion, green pepper
- eggplant, broccoli, cabbage, tomatoes
- mushrooms
- lettuce

0–10

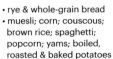

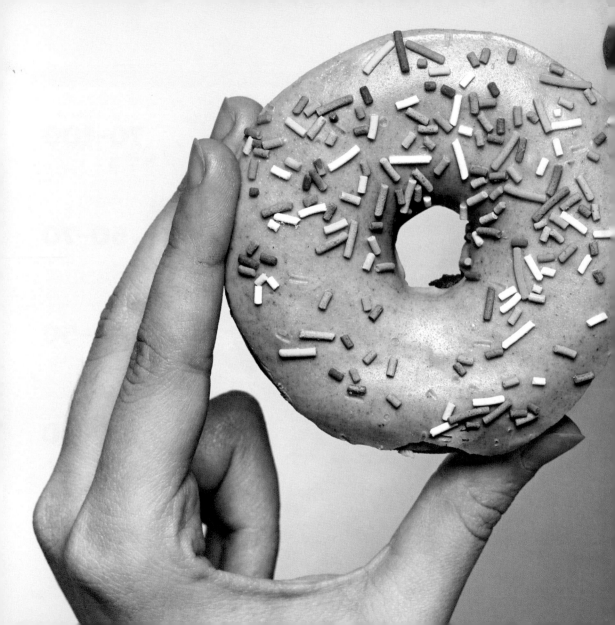

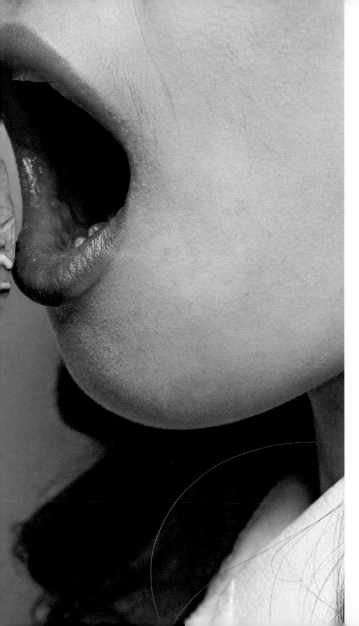

THE SWEET TOOTH QUIZ:

How Big Is Yours?

Okay, you know that consuming too much added sugar is bad for you. And yet it's in practically everything you eat, and you probably eat way more than you think. The next step is to figure out the patterns to your sugar consumption: Is it pretty much within acceptable limits, totally out of whack, or somewhere in between? This quiz is a powerful tool on your journey to understanding and limiting unwanted sugar intake.

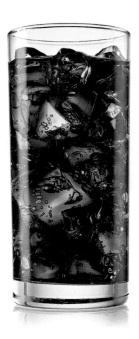
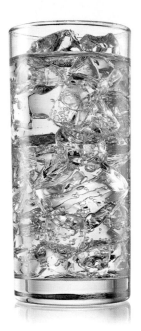
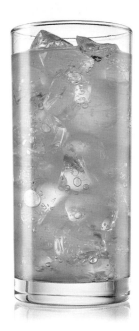

1 **How often do you eat or drink sugary foods or beverages (including ones made with artificial sweeteners)?**

A) Once or twice a month, at most. I'm not big on sweets.

B) I'll have dessert a couple of times per week, but I rarely drink regular or diet soda.

C) Pretty much every day.

2 **How much sugar or sweetener do you usually add to your coffee?**

A) None.

B) A teaspoon or one packet.

C) Two teaspoons or two packets. At least.

3 **What's your typical breakfast like?**

A) Scrambled eggs with vegetables, avocado toast, or even last night's leftovers.

B) Greek yogurt, oatmeal with fruit, or a smoothie.

C) Sugary cereal, a muffin, or a donut.

④ How often do you go out of your way to get something sugary—like stopping at the store just to buy candy?

A) Almost never.

B) Every once in a while, if I get a crazy craving for something.

C) Often—like, at least once a week.

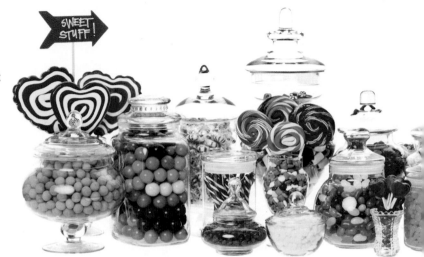

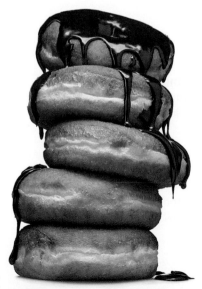

⑤ Do you ever eat sugary foods secretively?

A) No. If I'm having dessert, it's part of a meal or an event with others.

B) A couple of times a year, I definitely feel like polishing off a pint of ice cream on the couch by myself.

C) I usually wait to eat dessert until I'm alone, so I can really chow down without anyone judging me.

⑥ Do you hide sugary foods to eat them later?

A) No. Why would I do that?

B) Not usually. But if I know there's only one more piece of Aunt Milly's amazing pie left, I might rearrange a few things in the fridge to make it harder for anyone else to find.

C) Yup, I have a stash of my favorites to enjoy when I'm by myself.

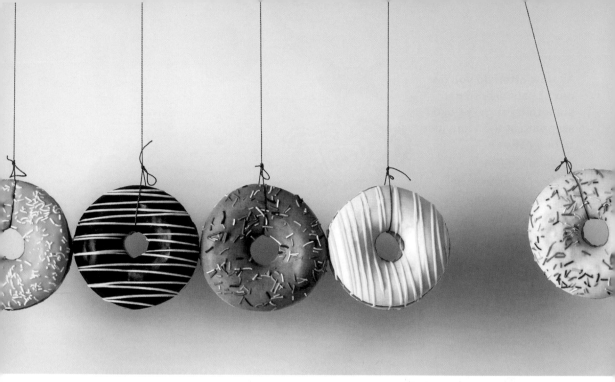

7 **Do you ever feel powerless in front of sugary foods or foods made with refined flour, like white bread or cookies?**

A) Rarely. It's just not my thing.

B) Maybe once in a while, if I'm starving. But usually I can have one or two cookies and stop.

C) Yes. Usually once I start eating stuff like that, it's really hard to stop. Even when I'm already full.

8 **While indulging, do you ever tell yourself that this is the "last time" you'll ever eat like this?**

A) No.

B) I tried once or twice in the past to cut out sugar, but I realized it wouldn't work in the long run.

C) I tell myself that a lot (and end up feeling bad when I don't follow through).

Know Your Sugar Score

Count up how many times you chose each letter (pages 26 to 28), then read the descriptions below to determine your sugar dependence and how *Sugar Shock* can help you move forward.

MOSTLY A'S Congrats! You don't have a sugar habit. However, you can still benefit from this book. *Sugar Shock* will reveal hundreds of everyday foods with hidden sugars that may have crept into your diet that you were unaware of—until now.

MOSTLY B'S You are in good command of your sugar intake, but this book will make you even wiser. You'll find hundreds of healthier swaps for surprisingly sugary foods, plus a treasure trove of low-sugar and sugar-free tips, so you'll stay on track.

MOSTLY C'S Sounds like sugar is a frequent choice for you, so you may be hooked. *Sugar Shock* is here to help. To jump-start your efforts to break free of sweets, turn the page to get smart about identifying added sugar on food labels.

NOW YOU'RE READY to learn exactly how much added sugar is in your diet with the 7-Day Sugar Tracker, page 46. Next, there's a 7-Day Sugar Step-Down Plan, page 70, to reduce your intake of added sugar, recalibrate your taste for sweet, and allow your body to adjust to the American Heart Association's daily recommended amount of added sugar. Then if you want to go even further, follow the 21-Day Sugar-Detox Meal Plan, page 83, to eliminate added sugar entirely for three weeks. Don't worry; there are lots of fruit and snacks! But the biggest perk of *Sugar Shock*? Our Smart Swaps—where we delve deep to expose the shocking amount of sugar in more than 100 common foods and share the practical fixes you'll need to conquer your cravings for sweet.

OLD LABEL

Nutrition Facts

Serving Size 2/3 cup (55g)
Servings Per Container About 8

Amount Per Serving

Calories 230	Calories from Fat 72

% Daily Value*

Total Fat 8g	**12**%
Saturated Fat 1g	**5**%
Trans Fat 0g	
Cholesterol 0mg	**0**%
Sodium 160mg	**7**%
Total Carbohydrate 37g	**12**%
Dietary Fiber 4g	**16**%
Sugars 12g	
Protein 3g	
Vitamin A	10%
Vitamin C	8%
Calcium	20%
Iron	45%

* Percent Daily Values are based on a 2,000 calorie diet.
Your daily value may be higher or lower depending on
your calorie needs.

	Calories:	2,000	2,500
Total Fat	Less than	65g	80g
Sat Fat	Less than	20g	25g
Cholesterol	Less than	300mg	300mg
Sodium	Less than	2,400mg	2,400mg
Total Carbohydrate		300g	375g
Dietary Fiber		25g	30g

NEW LABEL

Nutrition Facts

8 servings per container
Serving size   2/3 cup (55g)

Amount per serving

Calories   230

% Daily Value*

Total Fat 8g	**10**%
Saturated Fat 1g	**5**%
Trans Fat 0g	
Cholesterol 0mg	**0**%
Sodium 160mg	**7**%
Total Carbohydrate 37g	**13**%
Dietary Fiber 4g	**14**%
Total Sugars 12g	
Includes 10g Added Sugars	**20**%
Protein 3g	
Vitamin D 2mcg	10%
Calcium 260mg	20%
Iron 8mg	45%
Potassium 235mg	6%

* The % Daily Value (DV) tells you how much a nutrient in
a serving of food contributes to a daily diet. 2,000 calories
a day is used for general nutrition advice.

CHAPTER 3

SUGAR ON THE
LABEL

Read Between the Lines

To start limiting your sugar intake, take note of the added sugar line on the Nutrition Facts panel. This is a new addition by the Food and Drug Administration starting in 2020, and it will be in full effect by 2021. The total-sugar line includes both added sugars and sugars that occur naturally, such as in fruit or yogurt; the added-sugar line tells you the amount of sugar manufacturers used to enhance the product's flavor or texture. The Nutrition Facts panel also displays a percent daily value for added sugar and other nutrients. Don't get thrown off by it. This value is based on a higher added-sugar allowance than the American Heart Association's guidelines that are used throughout *Sugar Shock*. Because added sugar is associated with many health problems, we stuck with the lower limits. According to a study in the journal *Circulation*, the new added-sugar labeling policy may prevent hundreds of thousands of cases of diabetes and heart disease in the U.S. and could save $31 billion in healthcare costs over the next 20 years. Here are some other tips to note while reviewing the panel:

LOOK FOR WHERE SUGAR IS LISTED IN THE INGREDIENT LIST. Food ingredients are listed in order of volume, from highest to lowest amount.

DAILY VALUES ON THE LABEL ARE BASED ON A 2,000-CALORIE DIET. If you do not follow a 2,000-calorie diet or follow other dietary restrictions, this information should not be used as a guideline.

FOR FOODS THAT DO NOT CONTAIN A NUTRITION FACTS PANEL, websites like Calorie King or Food Data Central can help provide insight into the sugar content.

THERE ARE AT LEAST 57 DIFFERENT NAMES FOR ADDED SUGAR. To tell if a product contains added sugars, check the list of ingredients. First line of defense: Look out for any ingredient ending in "ose," such as maltose or sucrose. To help you further decode what's on the label, turn the page for the many aliases for added sugars.

Fifty Shades of Sugar

Here's all the ways sugar can show up in the food you eat, often in disguise!

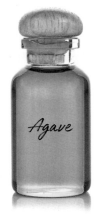

AGAVE NECTAR
(a.k.a. Agave Syrup)

FOUND IN: Cereals, ice cream, and organic foods

REASON TO AVOID: You'll use less because it's sweeter, but its sugar is more concentrated than even HCFS.

BARLEY MALT

FOUND IN: Beers, cereals, and candy bars

REASON TO AVOID: This grain-based sugar is half as sweet as white sugar, but it's just as high on the glycemic index.

BEET SUGAR

FOUND IN: More than 20 percent of the world's sugar

DON'T BE FOOLED: The word *beet* suggests this sugar is natural, but it's not. Beets are stripped of their other nutrients when processed into refined sugar, the form of added sugar in many packaged foods.

BLACKSTRAP MOLASSES

FOUND IN: Baked beans and gingerbread

REASON TO AVOID: While unsulfured blackstrap is high in antioxidants and nutrients such as iron, folate, and calcium, the sulfured kind is higher in empty calories and sulfur dioxide content. The label won't tell you which kind you're getting.

BROWN RICE SYRUP
(a.k.a. Rice Syrup or Rice Malt)

FOUND IN: Rice milk, cereal bars, and organic foods

DON'T BE FOOLED: Although brown rice syrup is touted as a healthy alternative to

HFCS, your body still processes it the same way.

BROWN SUGAR

FOUND IN: Baked goods, beverages, and sauces

DON'T BE FOOLED: Brown sugar is just as bad for you as table sugar. The only real difference is the taste and how it has been processed.

CANE JUICE (a.k.a. Evaporated Cane Juice)

FOUND IN: Yogurt, fruit juice, lemonade, and liquor (cachaça)

REASON TO AVOID: Cane juice is less processed than table sugar, so it retains more riboflavin, a nutrient that's naturally found in sugarcane. But because cane juice has the same chemical composition as table sugar, any benefit is negligible.

CANE JUICE CRYSTALS

FOUND IN: Yogurt, cake, cookies, and baked goods

DON'T BE FOOLED: Cane juice crystals are often presented as a healthy alternative to table sugar. This is fool's gold: It still contains all of the harmful properties of the white stuff.

CANE SUGAR

FOUND IN: 80 percent of the world's sugar

REASON TO AVOID: The vast majority of sugar from around the globe is manufactured from sugarcane, the world's largest crop. Studies have repeatedly shown how cane sugar drastically raises blood pressure and cholesterol and contributes to insulin resistance.

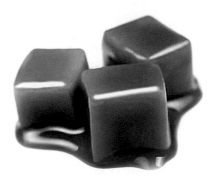

CARAMEL

FOUND IN: Sodas, desserts, and candy

REASON TO AVOID: It's made by heating various sugars, and it's high in both carbohydrates and calories.

CAROB SYRUP

FOUND IN: Cakes and cookies; used as a substitute for chocolate

REASON TO AVOID: When carob fruit is processed into syrup, the beneficial proteins and nutrients are stripped away, leaving mostly empty calories.

CASTER SUGAR
(a.k.a. Superfine Sugar)
FOUND IN: Baking products and mixed drinks

REASON TO AVOID: It's simply table sugar that's more finely granulated.

COCONUT SUGAR (a.k.a. Coconut Palm Sugar)
FOUND IN: Diabetic sweeteners and diabetic alternative foods

REASON TO AVOID: Coconut sugar ranks relatively low on the glycemic index and contains nutrients like potassium, magnesium, and iron. Even so, coconut sugar is still added sugar and negates its low glycemic or nutrient benefits.

CONFECTIONERS' SUGAR (see Powdered Sugar)

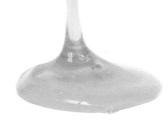

CORN SYRUP
FOUND IN: Sodas, fast food, and cookies

REASON TO AVOID: Corn syrup is 100 percent glucose, and just one tablespoon contains 16 grams of carbohydrates. For more information, see High-Fructose Corn Syrup (page 37).

CORN SYRUP SOLIDS
FOUND IN: Coffee creamers and dry beverage mixes

REASON TO AVOID: Composed mostly of a type of sugar called dextrose, you might think corn syrup solids are healthier than HFCS. Not so. Both are derived from the same product and are metabolized similarly by our bodies.

CRYSTALLINE FRUCTOSE
FOUND IN: Ice cream, baked goods, beverages; used as fruit flavoring

REASON TO AVOID: Crystalline fructose is essentially pure fructose and has been similarly linked to hyperlipidemia (high levels of fats in the blood) and fatty liver disease.

DATE SUGAR

FOUND IN: Baked goods and cookies

REASON TO AVOID: Made from chopped dates, this sugar is less processed but remains extremely high in sugar content. Every seven grams of date sugar has 1¾ teaspoons of the sweet stuff.

DEMERARA SUGAR

FOUND IN: Muffins and cakes; used as a sweetener in coffee and tea

REASON TO AVOID: This large-grained, textured sugar with caramel overtones has more nutrients than table sugar—but that's not saying much. Its trace amounts of proteins and vitamins are so insignificant they don't even appear on USDA food labels.

DEXTRIN

FOUND IN: Used as a food additive

REASON TO AVOID: This complex sugar is produced in our body when we break down starchy foods like baked goods. As a food additive, however, it often contains trace amounts of allergens such as wheat and corn.

DEXTROSE

FOUND IN: Sauces, cookies, cake mixes, candies, energy drinks, and frozen desserts

REASON TO AVOID: Dextrose has a high glycemic index, and most is made from genetically modified (GMO) corn.

DIASTATIC MALT POWDER

FOUND IN: Baked goods, milkshakes, ice cream, and flavored syrups

REASON TO AVOID: This powder is produced from barley and contains about two-thirds as many calories as table sugar.

DIASTASE

FOUND IN: Baked goods, beer, and honey

REASON TO AVOID: Diastase speeds up the process of transforming starches into maltose and, ultimately, glucose—types of sugar that contribute to blood sugar spikes.

ETHYL MALTOL

FOUND IN: Breads, cakes, and confectionary goods

REASON TO AVOID: This organic compound is often used as a flavoring due to its extremely sweet taste, which indicates its hazardously high sugar content.

EVAPORATED CANE JUICE

FOUND IN: Baked goods, cereals, and beverages

REASON TO AVOID: Evaporated cane juice is actually not a juice but rather a sweetener derived from sugar cane syrup. That means it's much more concentrated than a juice and has only trace amounts of nutrients.

FRUCTOSE

FOUND IN: Baked goods and soft drinks; naturally occurs in fruits and honey

REASON TO AVOID: Fructose consumption has been strongly linked to rising obesity rates in the past several decades, and research shows that fructose consumption, mostly from added sugars, now accounts for 10 percent of our daily caloric intake.

FRUIT JUICE CONCENTRATES

FOUND IN: Fruit juices and fruit-flavored yogurts

REASON TO AVOID: Juice concentrate is made by removing water from fruit juice, leaving out pulp and nutrients that would otherwise be found in naturally squeezed juice.

FRUIT SUGAR

FOUND IN: Dry mixes such as gelatin, pudding desserts, and powdered drinks

REASON TO AVOID: It's the same as table sugar, only it's been processed to have smaller, more uniformly sized crystals.

GALACTOSE

FOUND IN: Fast foods, vegetable products, and dairy products

REASON TO AVOID: Galactose is a naturally occurring sugar in some foods, like dairy, but it is also added to processed foods. When used in processed foods, it is known to cause blood sugar spikes that can drive up your blood pressure.

GLUCOSE

FOUND IN: Fruits, honey, fast foods, and baked goods

REASON TO AVOID: Glucose has the ability to raise the acidity of your blood and has been linked to high cholesterol, heart disease, and obesity.

GOLDEN SUGAR (a.k.a. Golden Caster Sugar and Unrefined Cane Sugar)

FOUND IN: Cake, biscuits, and meringues

REASON TO AVOID: Unrefined sugars like golden sugar retain some of the nutrients usually processed out, making them appear healthier. But just because it's incrementally better than refined sugar doesn't mean it's good for you.

GRAPE SUGAR
(see Glucose)

GRANULATED SUGAR
(see Sucrose)

HIGH-FRUCTOSE CORN SYRUP (HFCS)

FOUND IN: Fast foods, sodas, yogurts, canned foods, frozen pizzas, macaroni and cheese, cereal bars, and breads

REASON TO AVOID: To make HFCS, enzymes are added to corn syrup to convert some of its glucose to fructose. That makes HFCS "high" in fructose compared with the pure glucose that is in corn syrup. A study in the American Journal of Clinical Nutrition estimates that Americans eat 132 calories per day in high-fructose corn syrup. Your body metabolizes fructose in a way that encourages body-fat storage.

HONEY
(see Raw Honey)

FOUND IN: Baked goods and beverages

DON'T BE FOOLED: Honey is higher in fructose than table sugar, and pound for pound, its nutrients are about the same. Honey weighs more than the white stuff, so it's more caloric—there's 21 calories per teaspoon of honey versus 16 calories for table sugar. On the plus side, honey is sweeter than table sugar, so you don't need to use as much.

RAW HONEY

There is no FDA definition of raw honey, but it generally means that it hasn't been heated or filtered. There are claims that raw honey is better for you than processed or filtered honey because commercial honey has significantly less pollen. However, a study by the National Honey Board found that commercial processing of honey did not affect its nutrient content or antioxidant activity. Either way, they're both added sugar.

INVERT SUGAR
(a.k.a. Inverted Sugar)
FOUND IN: Candy, sodas, confectionary goods, and baked goods

REASON TO AVOID: Similar to high fructose corn syrup, except it's made from sugarcane or beets instead of corn. It's also produced through animal enzyme modification, a problem if you follow a vegan, vegetarian, kosher, or halal diet.

MALT SYRUP
FOUND IN: Bread, pastries, and diabetic alternative foods

REASON TO AVOID: Malt syrups have a high glycemic index and can therefore drastically raise blood sugar levels and increase sugar cravings.

MALTODEXTRIN
FOUND IN: Beer, sodas, candies, and processed foods

REASON TO AVOID: Nutrients like protein have been processed out of this common food additive. It's been found to be harmful to those who have celiac disease, wheat allergies, or corn allergies, because it's derived from corn.

MALTOSE
(a.k.a. Malt Sugar)
FOUND IN: Barley malt, beer, beverages, breakfast cereals, rice syrup, and corn syrup

REASON TO AVOID: It may be less sweet than table sugar, but maltose is used as a substitute for high-fructose corn syrup and is by no means a healthier variety of added sugar.

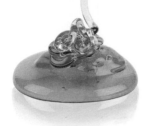

MAPLE SYRUP

FOUND IN: Used to top pancakes, waffles, and breakfast foods

REASON TO AVOID: Although it's less processed than other sugars, maple syrup is composed of mostly sucrose and contains minimal nutrients.

MOLASSES

FOUND IN: Gingerbread, cakes, cookies, and confectionary goods

REASON TO AVOID: While this syrup alternative to sugar is a good source of iron and calcium, it has laxative properties and can trigger allergies and asthma attacks due to its high sulfur content.

MUSCOVADO SUGAR

FOUND IN: Used as a sweetener in tea and coffee; a brown sugar replacement

REASON TO AVOID: A sibling to other brown sugars such as demerara and turbinado, muscovado sugar is less processed yet still contains five grams of carbs per teaspoon without any significant amounts of vitamins, minerals, or proteins. Claims of this being a "natural" brown sugar are misleading.

OAT SYRUP

FOUND IN: Granola bars, cereals, cookies, baked goods, and ice cream

REASON TO AVOID: While oat syrup is a good source of antioxidants, it's still high in both calories value and sugar content.

PANELA (a.k.a. Panocha)

FOUND IN: Baked goods and soft drinks

REASON TO AVOID: This sugar variety from Latin America is made from evaporated sugarcane juice and is basically pure sugar.

POWDERED SUGAR (a.k.a. Confectioners' Sugar or Icing Sugar)

FOUND IN: Cake decorations, icing, frosting, and baked goods

REASON TO AVOID: Confectioners' sugar contains 10 percent of your daily carbohydrate intake per ounce and is notorious for elevating blood sugar levels.

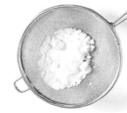

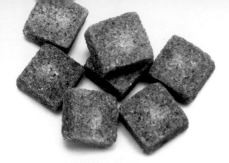

RAW SUGAR
(see *Turbinado Sugar*)

RICE SYRUP
FOUND IN: Pies, cookies, cakes, and granola bars
REASON TO AVOID: Rice syrup is relatively low on the glycemic index. However, it's extremely high in maltose, yet another sugar in disguise.

SORGHUM
FOUND IN: Cereals, cakes, muffins, beer, and alcoholic beverages
REASON TO AVOID: While a new generation of Southern chefs have made sorghum a trendy sweetener, it still contains sucrose, glucose, and fructose.

SORGHUM SYRUP
(a.k.a. *Sweet Sorghum*)
FOUND IN: Used as a topping for biscuits, grits, pancakes, and other breakfast foods
REASON TO AVOID: This version of sorghum is completely deficient of nutrients in any meaningful quantity.

SUCROSE (a.k.a. *Table Sugar, Granulated Sugar, White Sugar*)
FOUND IN: Cookies, cakes, biscuits, pies, and ice cream (to name a few)
REASON TO AVOID: A compound composed of half glucose and half fructose, sucrose has played a significant role in the growing instance of diabetes, obesity, and heart disease.

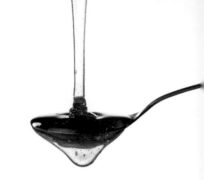

SYRUP
FOUND IN: Sodas, baked goods, breakfast foods, fast foods, and candy
REASON TO AVOID: All syrup products share common traits: high sugar content, loads of calories, and minimal nutritional values. U.S. labeling regulations prohibit imitation syrups—which are a combination of HFCS and caramel color—from having the word "maple" in their name. That's why these products are labeled "original syrup," "pancake syrup," "table syrup," and "waffle syrup."

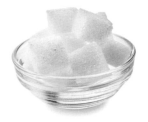

TABLE SUGAR
(See Sucrose)

TAPIOCA SYRUP
FOUND IN: Fruit drinks, health bars, and cereals
REASON TO AVOID: This syrup is often used as a healthy alternative to its maple counterpart, but the difference is minute. Although it has less sugar than maple syrup, it contains about the same number of calories.

TREACLE
FOUND IN: Tarts, meringues, and desserts
REASON TO AVOID: Made from the remains of brown sugar production, treacle is high in sucrose, fructose, and glucose.

TURBINADO SUGAR
(a.k.a. Raw Sugar)
FOUND IN: Baked goods; a replacement for white or brown sugar
REASON TO AVOID: Despite claims of its beneficial health effects, turbinado sugar is processed and metabolized in our bodies the same way as white sugar.

WHITE SUGAR
(See Sucrose)

YELLOW SUGAR
FOUND IN: Marshmallow Peeps, cookies, baked goods, and yellow frosting
REASON TO AVOID: The only difference between this and white or brown sugar is the color.

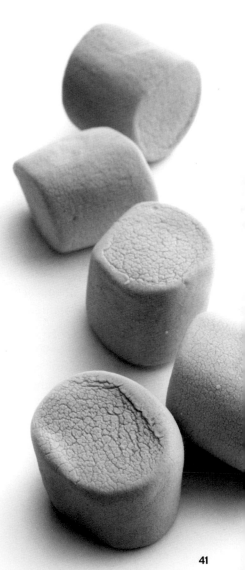

41

Fake News: Artificial Sweeteners

The theory behind artificial sweeteners is simple: If you use them instead of sugar, you get the joy of sweet-tasting beverages and foods without the downer of extra calories, potential weight gain, and their related health issues. According to a survey from Mintel, a consumer research firm, 61 percent of women in the U.S. use artificial sweeteners daily, and 50 percent drink diet soda. The three biggies—saccharin, aspartame, and sucralose—contain hardly any calories and are sweeter than sweet. Yet there's growing concern in the scientific community that fake sugars might be doing more harm than good. Here's what's inside those packets of pink, blue, and yellow.

SACCHARIN (a.k.a. Sweet'n Low) This sweetener was discovered in 1879 and is the result of a chemical reaction that produces methyl anthranilate. It has only ⅛ calorie per teaspoon versus sugar's 15, yet it's 300 times sweeter than the natural stuff. The downside of saccharin—used in toothpastes like Colgate and Crest and the diet soda Tab—is its bitter chemical aftertaste.

ASPARTAME (a.k.a. Equal or Nutrasweet) Slightly less bitter-tasting than saccharin, aspartame is derived from the amino acids L-aspartic acid and L-phenylalanine. Available since 1981, aspartame contains 24 calories per teaspoon, but because it's 180 times sweeter than sugar, a little goes a long way: A 12-ounce can of Diet Coke supplies less than 1 calorie from aspartame, while the high-fructose corn syrup in Coca-Cola Classic packs 100 calories.

SUCRALOSE (a.k.a. Splenda) This sweetener is made from sugar and tastes the closest to the real thing. To create it, food chemists substitute chlorine atoms for three hydrogen-oxygen groups on the sucrose molecule. That switch makes Splenda a tongue-tingling 600 times sweeter than sugar.

The AHA and the American Diabetes Association (ADA) have given a cautious nod to artificial sweeteners to help reduce added sugar in your diet. Yet, the effects of the fake stuff remains a hot topic as Americans continue consuming artificial sweeteners and the rate of obesity skyrockets. A study in the *International Journal of Obesity* suggests that when we offer our bodies diet drinks but give them no calories, they crave real sugar even more. "Substitutes may not signal the same satiety hormones as sugar, making it easier to overeat," says Lona Sandon, RD, an assistant professor at the University of Texas Southwestern Medical Center. It's also possible that these products change the way we taste food, according to David Ludwig, MD, PhD, an obesity and weight-loss specialist at Boston Children's Hospital. People who routinely use artificial sweeteners may find less intensely sweet foods, such as fruit, less appealing and unsweetened foods, such as vegetables, unpalatable.

IS STEVIA HEALTHIER THAN
FAKE SUGAR?

Stevia is one of the few no-calorie plant-based sweeteners. Like honey, it's referred to as a "natural" sweetener; however, the FDA has no formal definition for "natural." Research suggests Stevia may assist in reducing blood glucose following a meal and improve insulin response. Stevia is considered safe by the ADA, but "in appropriate amounts." So while Stevia may be better than the fake stuff, it's best used in moderation.

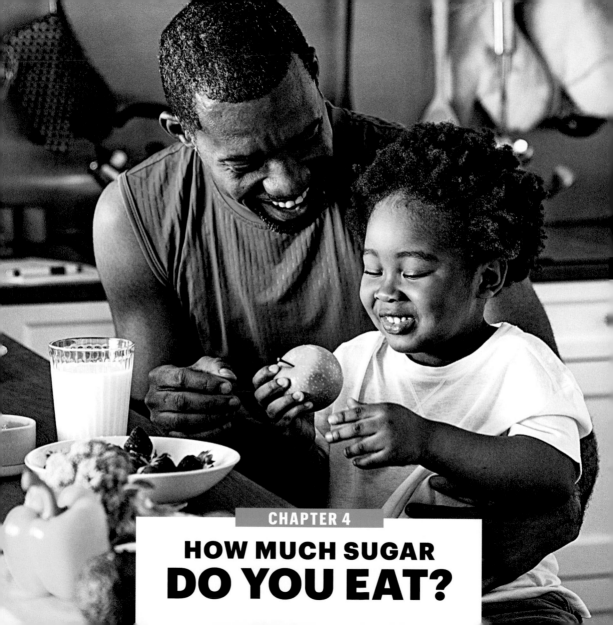

CHAPTER 4

HOW MUCH SUGAR DO YOU EAT?

Get a Grip on Sugar

The 7-Day Sugar Tracker (next page) will become a vital tool to help you understand your food choices and eating patterns and how they relate to the amount of sugar you eat. Armed with this powerful knowledge, you'll have the awareness it takes to help cut back on your sugar consumption.

For the next week, use the 7-Day Sugar Tracker to record how much added sugar you eat every day. You'll note the food you consume, the portion size and sugar content, the situation or meal when you ate it, and your feelings or mood at the time. The tracker will quickly expose the amount of added sugar in your diet—and the results could shock you. The amount of sugar adds up so fast! You'll also start to notice habits like when you mindlessly reach for sugar, the daily run for latte and muffins, your trips to the office vending machine for a granola bar, or when you eat because you're feeling bored. Make sure to write down the details of your meal as soon as possible after eating. Research shows that people tend to be less accurate the longer they wait to record.

The 7-Day Sugar Tracker

It's one thing to keep track of added sugar when you are in control, such as when you're baking treats for the fam or adding a teaspoon of sugar to your coffee or tea. But nutrition labels on foods you buy from the supermarket show sugar amounts in grams, not teaspoons. Don't let that confuse you! As you start to keep track of your daily sugar consumption, you can simply add up the grams. **If you are more comfortable keeping track by teaspoons, then simply divide the number of grams by four. If you want to keep track in grams, them simply multiply the teaspoons by four. Because the FDA's new nutrition label rule is not yet in full effect, some products may list only "Total Sugar" instead of "Added Sugar." While total sugar also includes natural sugar, the tracker will still help you identify the major sources of sugar in your diet.**

HERE'S HOW TO GET STARTED: Let's say you had a flavored yogurt for breakfast on Day 1, like in the example at right. Using the tracker, note the food item, the size of the container, the sugar amount, the situation or time of day, and your feelings or mood at the time. Continue to fill in each row throughout the day and be sure to include any beverages or snacks. You don't need to include fresh fruits or foods that do not contain added sugar. At the end of your day, fill in the total amount of sugar and calculate the total teaspoons or the total grams—whichever is easier for you. Continue for the rest of the week, adding up the daily totals as you go and comparing them to the recommended limits of added sugar by the AHA:

Daily limit for women:
24 grams / 6 teaspoons

Daily limit for men:
36 grams / 9 teaspoons

Daily limit for kids: (ages 2-18)
No more than 6 teaspoons / 24 grams

1 TSP = 4 GRAMS

BY THE END OF THE WEEK, you may be shocked by how much sugar you eat. To start cutting back, target foods with high sugar content and swap them out. Plus, look for recurring situations and moods associated with eating sugary foods so you can start to break those patterns.

Example

Food	Portion Amount	Sugar Amount	Situation/Time	Feelings/Mood
Flavored Yogurt	5.3 oz	15 g	Breakfast/ ate at desk	A little hungry
Ketchup	1 Tbsp	4 g	Lunch on burger	Ravenous
Hamburger bun	1	3 g	Lunch with burger	Ravenous
Frappuccino	9½ oz	32 g	Afternoon	Needed a pick-me-up
Crackers	5	2 g	Before dinner with cheese	Late start to dinner, feeling hungry
Frozen chicken Parmesan	1 package	4 g	Dinner	Too tired to cook

DAY 1: Total sugar 60 grams   *Significantly higher than the recommended maximum!*

Day 1

Food	Portion Amount	Sugar Amount	Situation/Time	Feelings/Mood

Food	Portion Amount	Sugar Amount	Situation/Time	Feelings/Mood

DAY 1: Total sugar _____

Day 2

Food	Portion Amount	Sugar Amount	Situation/Time	Feelings/Mood

Food	Portion Amount	Sugar Amount	Situation/Time	Feelings/Mood

DAY 2: **Total sugar** _____

Day 3

Food	Portion Amount	Sugar Amount	Situation/Time	Feelings/Mood

Food	Portion Amount	Sugar Amount	Situation/Time	Feelings/Mood

DAY 3: **Total sugar** _____

Day 4

Food	Portion Amount	Sugar Amount	Situation/Time	Feelings/Mood

Food	Portion Amount	Sugar Amount	Situation/Time	Feelings/Mood

DAY 4: **Total sugar** _____

Day 5

Food	Portion Amount	Sugar Amount	Situation/Time	Feelings/Mood

Food	Portion Amount	Sugar Amount	Situation/Time	Feelings/Mood

DAY 5: **Total sugar** _____

Day 6

Food	Portion Amount	Sugar Amount	Situation/Time	Feelings/Mood

Food	Portion Amount	Sugar Amount	Situation/Time	Feelings/Mood

DAY 6: **Total sugar** _____

Day 7

Food	Portion Amount	Sugar Amount	Situation/Time	Feelings/Mood

Food	Portion Amount	Sugar Amount	Situation/Time	Feelings/Mood

DAY 7: **Total sugar** _____

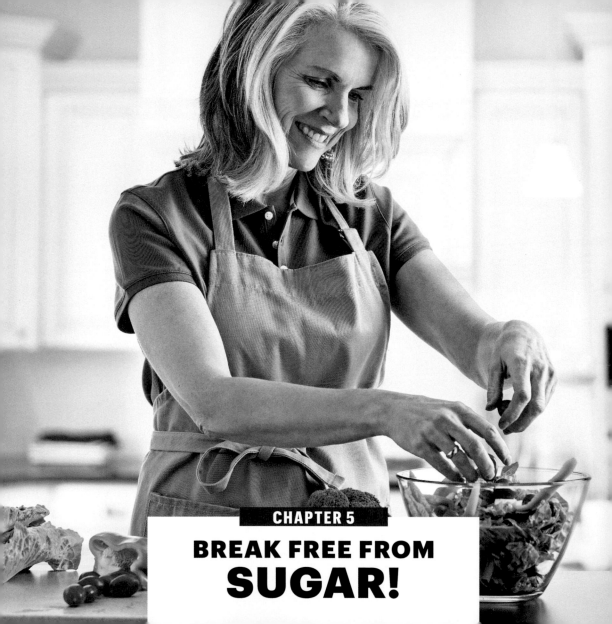

CHAPTER 5

BREAK FREE FROM
SUGAR!

Clean Up Your Diet

Get ready to break the hold that sugar has on your body. We'll get you ready for a Simple 7-Day Sugar Step-Down Plan (page 70) to help you wean yourself from added sugar in an easy and meaningful way. Then, if you want to go further, the 21-Day Sugar-Detox Meal Plan (page 83) will eliminate added sugar completely from your diet for three weeks. The ultimate goal of all this sweet sacrifice? Once you learn to manage your intake of added sugar, it will be easy to adhere to AHA limits—without feeling deprived. That adds up to a winning strategy to ensure long-term, low-sugar diet success.

Don't expect perfection. If you do give in to a craving, don't blame yourself or throw in the towel. Recognize how omnipresent sugar is, making it hard to avoid. Get back on track and don't sweat it!

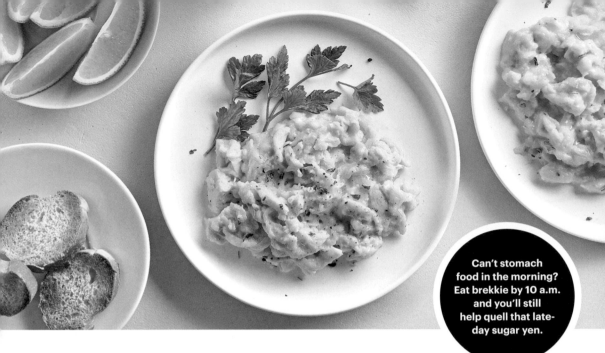

Can't stomach food in the morning? Eat brekkie by 10 a.m. and you'll still help quell that late-day sugar yen.

9 Ways to Outwit Sugar

To prepare for the 7-Day Sugar Step-Down Plan (page 70), get familiar with these nine simple strategies, each of which addresses a small but crucial component of achieving freedom from added sugar. Some will guide you toward eating the right foods, and others are designed to help you find satisfaction without turning to sugar.

1. BEGIN YOUR DAY WITH BREAKFAST— AND PACK IT WITH PROTEIN. Research shows that eating breakfast is common among people who have lost weight and kept it off. But when it comes to controlling sugar, what you eat is important. If you start your day with quickly digested simple carbs—a bowl of cereal (even whole-grain), a bagel, a muffin, or excess fruit that is easily

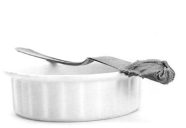

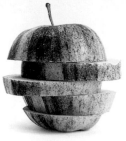

overconsumed such as grapes, watermelon, or pineapple—then poof! Your blood sugar levels will spike and drop precipitously, leaving you ravenous within hours. The fix? Pump up the protein, which slows digestion. Think options like moderate amounts of plain Greek yogurt and cheese, peanut or other nut butters, and eggs. Studies show that calorie for calorie, protein is more filling than carbohydrates or fat. Plus, MRI scans of high-protein breakfast eaters in a University of Missouri study showed reduced activity in areas of the brain associated with cravings.

2. NEVER GO HUNGRY.

Meal skipping is a guaranteed way to fire up sugar cravings. This lowers blood sugar levels and causes you to overeat later in the day to make up for missed calories. Keep things steady by eating five times a day—three meals and two snacks. Enjoy nourishing whole foods such as whole grains, beans, lean meats such as poultry, fish, nuts, unsweetened low-fat dairy, eggs, and veggies. They'll fill you up and give you the ideal balance of essential nutrients to steady your blood sugar and insulin levels and extinguish cravings for sugar.

3. STAY HYDRATED.

A study in the *Journal of Human Nutrition and Dietetics* found that adults who increased their daily intake of water also reduced their daily intake of sugar and calories. Water helps increase feelings of satiety, which can help prevent overeating as well as replace sugary beverages. There are many ways to drink more water: Have a glass when you wake up in the morning and with every meal, and keep a filled glass or water bottle beside you throughout the day. If you'd like, you can add fresh cucumber slices, mint, or a slice of citrus to your water. Also, be sure to include water-rich food like fruits and veggies in your diet.

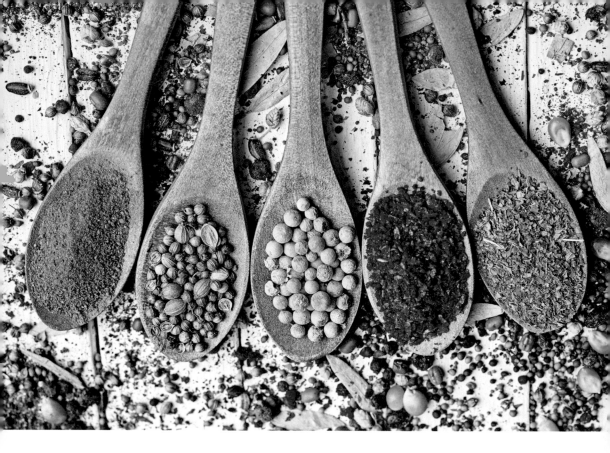

4. JOLT YOUR TASTE BUDS WITH FLAVOR, NOT SUGAR. Sugar always tastes the same. On the other hand, herbs, spices, and other add-ins offer wonderfully diverse and surprising flavors. If you've ever seeded a fragrant vanilla bean for a dish or topped a sliced tomato with fresh basil leaves, you know what a taste punch these ingredients deliver. Experiment with herbs and spices (see page 78), and don't forget other flavor boosters like balsamic vinegar, extra-virgin olive oil, lemon and orange zest, roasted peppers, hot sauce, and toasted nuts, to name a few.

5. SLEEP MORE, CRAVE LESS.
Another key to stopping sugar cravings is balancing the hormones ghrelin (an appetite trigger) and leptin (which signals satiety), along with insulin. Get these hormones working in harmony and you'll experience fewer cravings—and less fat storage. But if you get less than the recommended seven to nine hours of sleep, you may be undercutting this goal. In a University of Chicago study, a few sleepless nights were enough to drop levels of leptin by 18 percent and boost levels of ghrelin by about 30 percent.

Those two changes alone caused cravings for sugary foods to jump 45 percent. Sleep deprivation not only makes sugary foods more appealing but may also lower your ability to resist them. According to research at the University of California at Berkeley, the parts of your brain that usually put the brakes on cravings aren't as active when you're tired.

6. MOVE AWAY FROM CRAVINGS. If you're plagued by strong cravings for sugar, getting your body moving may help deactivate them. According to a study in *Applied Psychology, Nutrition, and Metabolism*, the more you sit, the greater your appetite—even if your body doesn't need the calories. Moderate exercise also helps keep muscle cells sensitive to insulin. Strength training builds stronger muscles, which in turn use up more glucose. Any physical activity that you enjoy will help get sugar off your brain.

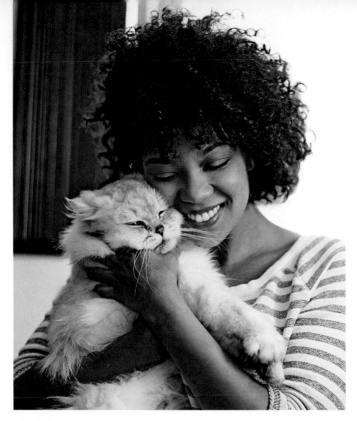

8. FIND HEALTHY WAYS TO BOOST YOUR MOOD. We often reach for sugar when we're stressed, lonely, or bored. But there are better ways to turn around a bad mood or energy lull. Make a list of activities that you can whip out any time you find yourself reaching for sweets. The sugar-free happiness builders you choose should be things that are accessible and elicit the same pleasure you feel when you indulge in a dessert. Think of things you can do instantly and that last for 15–20 minutes. For instance: Listen to music, dance like crazy, call a friend, paint your toenails, go for a bike ride, play with your cat, watch trashy TV, plan a dream vacation, or read a book.

7. BREAK SUGAR'S EMOTIONAL HOLD. The first step toward breaking the strong connection between emotions and food is to become aware of the feelings that drive you to crave sweets. (To help, go to the 7-Day Sugar Tracker, page 46). In those moments, remember this simple but powerful mantra: "Stop. Slow down. Think." It will help you determine whether you really want the sweet or are just feeding your emotions.

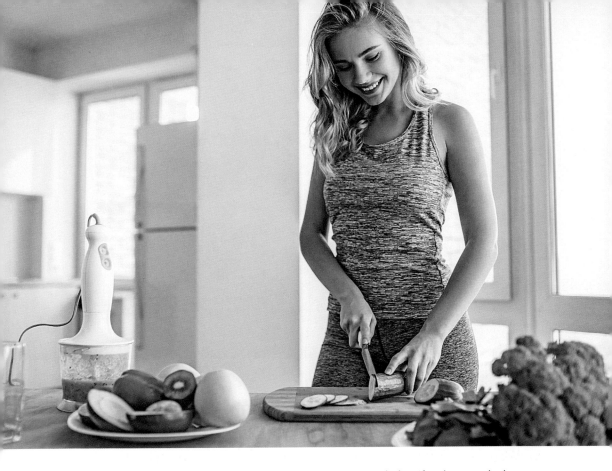

9. PINPOINT YOUR SUGAR PITFALLS. Think through your day and identify where and when you are most susceptible to sugar's lure, then ask yourself why you "need" sugar in those moments. Is it because you're starving when you get to work and the doughnuts in the break room are just too tempting to resist? Empower yourself with new, positive alternatives you can use to meet that need. Have 10–15 nuts or ¼ cup of cut-up fruit on hand when a craving strikes (and check out our healthy snack ideas, page 238).

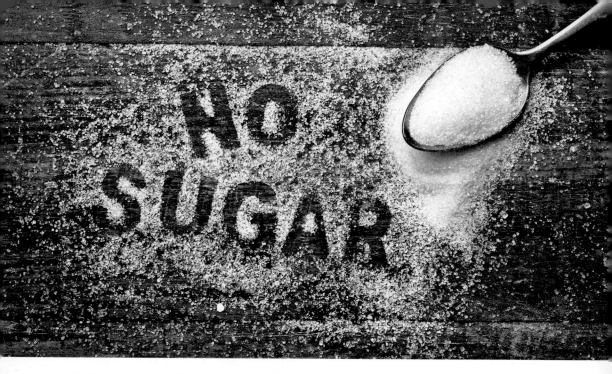

7-Day Sugar Step-Down Plan

Over the next week, you'll start to break the hold sugar has on your body by gradually eliminating sources of added sugar in your diet. The goal of this plan is to help you establish a healthier relationship with sugar, not to deprive you of sweets forever. Yes, this plan many seem like a challenge at first, but we've included plenty of tips and strategies to help. In as little as one week, you can begin to train your taste buds to stop craving foods loaded with added sugar.

As you go through this plan, refer to the 7-Day Sugar Tracker (page 46), that you have filled out, as it provided you with essential data about your eating behavior. This way you can pinpoint which sugar step-down strategies work best for you. Here's how to get started.

MONDAY

Nix the Snacking Sweets

Start off by ditching the brownies, the office candy stash, and your coworker's birthday cake. That low-fat blueberry muffin and the "nutritious" energy bar you stashed in your purse have also got to go. It's a no-brainer place to start because the sugar in sweets is easy to spot. Plus, you'll slash a whole bunch of unnecessary calories from your diet while you're at it.

When you notice a sugar craving, stop and take a moment to figure out what's really going on. Addressing what's truly driving the urge to eat sugar sets you up for success. Here are the top contenders:

YOUR BLOOD SUGAR IS TOO LOW. That means you're skipping meals or spacing them out too much, or you're not eating enough blood sugar-steadying protein.
Sugar Swap: Pair a sugary snack with protein—like mixed nuts and no-sugar-added dried fruit. The healthy fats in the nuts slow absorption of the fruit's natural sugars so you get back into balance and cravings stop. When you do have a meal, add grilled chicken or chickpeas to that pasta salad.

YOU'RE TIRED. As in, you're short on sleep.
Sugar Swap: Caffeinate with coffee or tea instead of a soda; take a brief walk, or take a nap.

YOU'RE HAVING PMS OR ARE IN PERIMENOPAUSE. Inadequate levels of progesterone or estrogen trigger cravings for sweets by cutting the feel-good brain chemicals serotonin, dopamine, and norepinephrine, which leads to insomnia, headaches, fatigue, or mild depression.
Sugar Swap: Try eating edamame, because soy contains compounds called isoflavones that mimic estrogen in the body. If that doesn't curb the sugar cravings, go for nature's sweet treats—an orange, a handful of berries, carrot sticks, or a small baked sweet potato.

Stop Reaching for Sugar Automatically

Any time you would normally use sugar or artificial sweetener, notice your impulse and then hold back. Be mindful of your use of so-called "natural" sweeteners like agave or honey—your body handles those the same way as other sugars. Eat your oatmeal minus that sprinkle of brown sugar on top (add ¼ of a sliced banana instead) and take your coffee with a shake of cinnamon instead of flavored syrup. Eliminating added sugar might leave your taste buds yearning for sweetness. Instead, get your sweet fix in with these creative hacks:

ADD VANILLA EXTRACT. While it's not actually sweet, vanilla reminds us of ice cream, cake, and other desserts. Add a few drops—or the contents of a vanilla bean—to tea, yogurt, oatmeal, nut butters, or smoothies.

TRY TOASTED UNSWEETENED COCONUT. These flakes are naturally sweet and add nuttiness and crunch to breakfast or dessert. Opt for the large flakes over tiny shreds; more surface area means more flavor on your tongue.

CARAMELIZE ONIONS. If you're making tomato sauce or soup, skip the sugar and caramelize any onions in the recipe instead of just sautéing them. Their natural sweetness subs in well.

CREATE CONTRAST WITH SALT. Because sugar and salt are polar opposites, a dash of salt can intensify sweetness. Try it on foods that are naturally a little sweet, like sweet potatoes, butternut squash soup, or sliced fruit.

It's best to avoid using the word *can't* during this plan. Instead of telling yourself, "I can't eat that" when faced with temptation, think, "I don't eat that." The former feels like you're punishing yourself, while the later feels empowering.

WEDNESDAY
Give Up Sugary Drinks

You know soda has added sugar, and so does a vanilla-flavored coffee drink. But the sugar in other drinks might not be so obvious, like coconut water (some brands add sugar), bottled iced teas, flavored waters, and even artificially sweetened drinks. (For more on sweetened drinks, see Chapter 6, page 90.) Chances are, you have firsthand experience with how hard it is to leave behind the caffeine high, the sweet jolt, and the comforting ritual of popping open a can. Take heart: Most people can't just drop a habit like soda; they need to replace it. To help you stick to your commitment to ditch sugary drinks, make it a point to avoid sugar triggers in the first place. Think about it this way: If your soda jones is a caffeine thing, switch to unsweetened coffee, tea, or dark chocolate. If stepping out for an afternoon latte is all about boredom, make things less dreary. Walk over to a coworker's office for a chat instead.

THURSDAY

Go Plain

Start reading ingredient labels like it's your job. Some flavored fruit yogurts, cereals, and prepared oatmeal pack nearly six teaspoons of added sugar per serving, which is the maximum amount of added sugar the AHA recommends for women in an entire day. Sweeten your favorite foods with whole fruit instead. Be on the lookout: Dressings, pasta sauces, crackers, ketchup, and soups are also common sources of hidden sugar.

FRIDAY

Kick Out Refined Grains

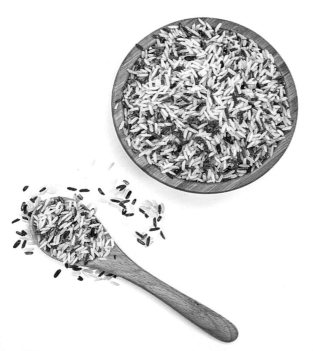

Consider refined grains (i.e., white flour, white rice, and white bread) basically just sugar in the form of simple carbohydrates. In fact, you might not think you have a sweet tooth, but if you're eating bagels and pasta on a regular basis, you're probably fooling yourself, according to nutritionist Brooke Albert. "Pizza is basically dessert. Your body consumes it just like a slice of cake," she says. The fix: Eat carbs, but make them whole-grain. Brown rice, sprouted-grain bread, and quinoa are all your friends. (See page 76 to gauge the healthiest carb choices.)

SATURDAY

Watch the Booze

Red wine may have phytochemicals and health benefits, but the truth is that when we drink alcohol, it turns to sugar in our bodies. If you decide to have a drink, stick to a 12-ounce light beer, a small glass of wine, or one shot of distilled spirits (vodka, gin, rum, Scotch, bourbon) sans mixers. Most mixers—even tonic waters—have added sugar or are fruit juice–based, so avoid those. (For more on cocktails, see page 139.)

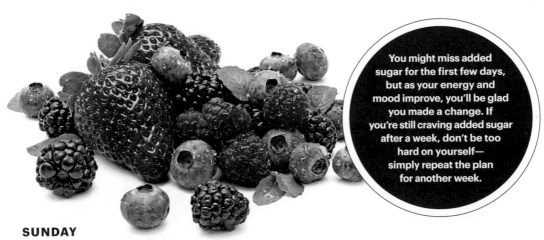

You might miss added sugar for the first few days, but as your energy and mood improve, you'll be glad you made a change. If you're still craving added sugar after a week, don't be too hard on yourself— simply repeat the plan for another week.

SUNDAY

Celebrate with Fruit

By today, you've reset your taste buds for less sweetnees. Take a moment to notice how your usual sliced banana with cereal or the apple in your brown-bag lunch now tastes sweeter. Continue to enjoy fruit for snacks or add it to main dishes and salads whenever you can. Whole fruit also packs fiber, vitamins, and water that keep you feeling satisfied.

EAT RARELY
Refined Grains

WHAT YOU'RE EATING Processed grains like white bread and pasta, cookies, cakes, and pastries have been stripped of fiber and valuable nutrients such as antioxidants and speed through your gut, making you hungry shortly after eating them.

BEST AMOUNT The 2015–2020 Dietary Guidelines for Americans recommends eating six ounces of grain foods daily (based on a 2000-calorie diet) with no more than half (or three ounces) of that grain intake from refined grains. However, due to the possible detrimental effects of consuming mostly refined grains, the Harvard T. H. Chan School recommends choosing mostly whole grains. Have no more than two handfuls of refined grains daily. If you can't give up these carbs right away, try to eat them with protein to help decelerate their race through your stomach.

EAT IN MODERATION
Whole Grains

WHAT YOU'RE EATING Your body requires more energy to process whole grains like unprocessed brown, red, or black rice, and quinoa. It can't process whole grains as quickly as refined grains, and because of this, you'll experience greater satiety and fewer cravings.

BEST AMOUNT Eat up to three servings a day of 100 percent whole grains. People who do so are 76 times more likely to get the most fiber—which has been linked with weight loss.

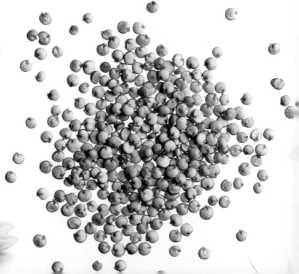

EAT YOUR FILL
Starches

WHAT YOU'RE EATING Research reveals a welcome twist on this group of foods: It's not carbs like corn or potatoes that do waistline damage, but the way in which they are prepared (fried in oil versus baked) and the portions in which they are eaten.

BEST AMOUNT Natural sugary foods like potatoes, corn, or bananas that contain resistant starch (i.e., starch that is resistant to digestion) can show waist-slimming promise when consumed with lower sugary foods. Evidence from the British Nutrition Foundation suggests that resistant starch acts like fiber, slowing digestion, shutting down hunger hormones, and increasing calorie burn.

EAT YOUR FILL
Legumes

WHAT YOU'RE EATING Even though they contain protein and fiber, beans and peas have been banished from a lot of diet plans. In fact, they should be your go-to carbs. One analysis found that people felt 31 percent fuller after eating about 1 cup of legumes daily.

BEST AMOUNT Try swapping in a ¼ cup of cooked beans for an ounce of ground beef in burgers; you'll save nearly four grams of fat and 30 calories. Then work beans and other legumes like peanuts and chickpeas into your regular meals.

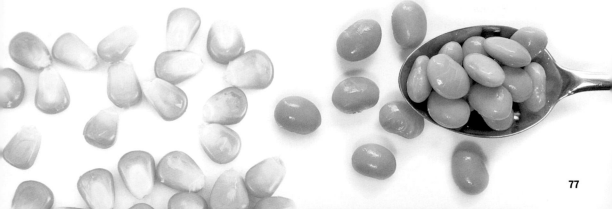

Spice Up Your Life!

Now that you've trained your taste buds to stop craving foods loaded with sugar, it's time to discover how herbs and spices can jazz up your meals instead of sweeteners. Here are our favorite flavor enhancers and how to use them.

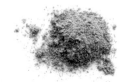

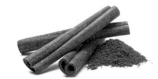

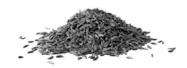

CARDAMOM

This sweet member of the ginger family can help stabilize blood sugar and has been linked to a significant reduction in blood pressure. Green cardamom, whole or ground, is the variety used most often in cooking.

Cardamom gives a lift to baked goods such as muffins and savory dishes like rice and curries. For an aromatic rice dish, add cracked cardamom pods to water before boiling or use ground cardamom to season after cooking.

CINNAMON

One of the most common healthy replacements for sugar, cinnamon helps blunt the rise in blood sugar that can occur when you eat a carbohydrate-rich meal. Whole cinnamon sticks release their flavor slowly when heated, while ground cinnamon makes its impact immediately.

Cinnamon enhances curries, baked goods, and fruit. Toss diced apples with walnuts, dried cranberries, and ground cinnamon for a healthy snack.

CUMIN

With its musky, peppery flavor and citrusy aroma, this spice can stimulate enzymes necessary for healthy digestion. Lightly toasting the seeds in a dry skillet before grinding them in a mini food processor brings out the flavor in their oils.

Cumin compliments lentils, beans, and other legumes. Stir ground cumin into hummus with lemon juice.

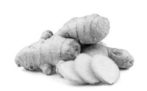

GINGER

In both its fresh and dried forms, this spice can help soothe an upset stomach and nausea. While ground ginger has a milder taste than the root, either will add a warm, sweetly spiced flavor to a wide variety of dishes.

Baked goods, salad dressings, and beverages benefit from ginger. Add a one-inch piece of peeled fresh ginger or one teaspoon of ground ginger to a smoothie.

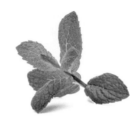

MINT

If you're used to having something sweet after meals, mint is a great substitute. This herb aids digestion and reduces your risk for post-meal bloating. There are more than 600 varieties, but spearmint and peppermint are used most often in cooking and make a refreshing addition to both sweet and savory dishes.

Citrus is the perfect companion to mint. For a healthy dessert, top orange slices with fresh mint and toasted coconut flakes.

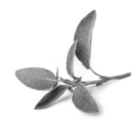

SAGE

A little sage goes a long way. This bold herb adds an earthy flavor and fragrance to foods. It may also help boost brain health, lower LDL ("bad") cholesterol, and raise HDL ("good") cholesterol. Because sage is similar botanically to rosemary, the herbs are often paired in recipes.

Sage works well with roasts because it can withstand long cooking times, and it pairs particularly well with pork and poultry.

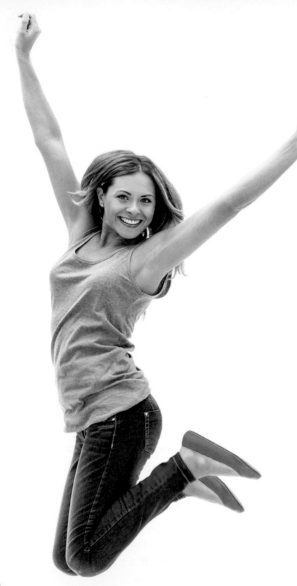

FIVE FABULOUS BODY BENEFITS

If you've successfully completed the 7-Day Sugar Step-Down Plan (page 70), congratulations! Soon you will start to see these wonderfully positive effects on your body. (If you haven't done the step-down plan yet or are ready to embark on the 21-Day Sugar-Detox Meal Plan, page 83, let these benefits inspire you to get started.)

1. YOUR HEART WILL DO A HAPPY DANCE.
Once you're able to reduce your added sugar intake to AHA-recommended levels, your risk of dying from heart-related illness may plummet as much as threefold, according to research at St. Luke's Mid-Atlantic Heart Institute. Within a few weeks' time, you might see a 10 percent decrease in LDL cholesterol and a 20 to 30 percent decrease in triglycerides. Your blood pressure will decrease too.

2. YOUR FACE WILL THANK YOU. Systemic inflammation is a known acne trigger, and sugar is inflammatory. One study in the American Journal of Clinical Nutrition found that when non–soda drinkers consumed one 12-ounce can a day for three weeks, their inflammation levels increased by 87 percent.

3. YOU WON'T HAVE TO FAKE A SMILE. It's normal to be cranky after you've ditched sweets. (After all, you've relied on sugary foods for comfort and a quick hit of energy.) But once you're over your sugar fix, you'll feel better than ever. A Columbia University study found that women who eat a diet high in sugar and refined grains are more likely to experience anxiety, irritability, and mood swings.

4. YOU'LL REMEMBER THE NAME OF YOUR PARTNER'S BOSS. Battling brain fog? Sugar may be to blame. One animal study at UCLA concluded that a diet high in added sugar hinders learning and memory. The study shows that over time, eating lots of sugar may actually damage communication among your brain cells.

5. YOU'LL PROBABLY LOSE THOSE EXTRA 10 POUNDS. While you replace those sugary calories with foods that contain less added sugar, you probably won't be eating more calories overall. Scaling back your sugar habit by just 200 calories a day could help you drop 10 pounds in five to six months.

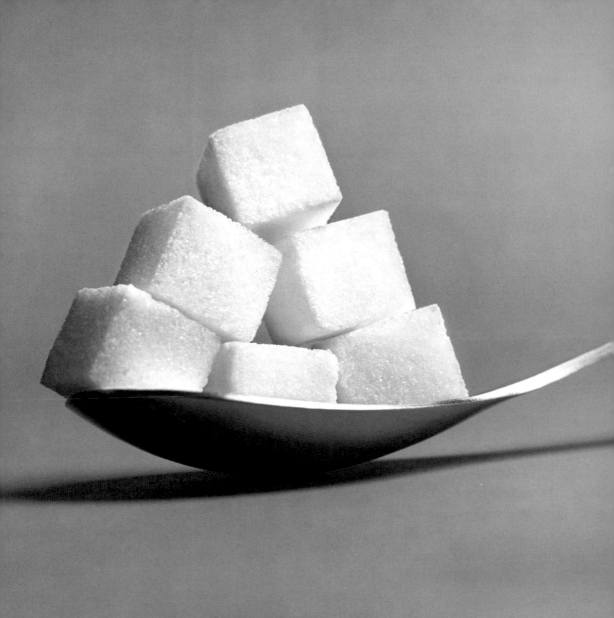

21-Day Sugar-Detox Meal Plan

Ready to eliminate added sugar from your diet? This detox plan was created to offer loads of flavor without a single sugar crash. That's right: For three weeks, you'll have a delicious diet completely free of added sugar, and you may not even notice it's gone.

THIS PLAN will help simplify your sugar detox transition. The meals are packed with healthy fats, fiber, and protein, all of which help keep you satiated throughout the day. This is important because the sweet stuff is one of the first things many people crave when they're hungry (see Your Body on Sugar, page 16), and these nutrients are critical to helping you stay on track.

During this detox, try to abstain from all added sugar. When using packaged products for these meals—such as sprouted-grain breads, wraps, pasta sauces, salad dressings, ketchup, and soups—examine the labels to identify hidden added sugars (see Fifty Shades of Sugar, page 32). Use the Smart Swaps throughout the book to locate approved products.

Naturally sweet fresh fruit is used to help you progress through the detox. Use the fruit chart (page 000) to find seasonal swaps. Additionally, an abundance of fiber-rich veggies will help you stay full; cook them any way you like, such as steamed and flavored with Greek or Italian seasoning, curry or garlic powder, fresh lemon, or a sprinkle of grated Parmesan cheese. Or roast or sauté them in extra-virgin olive oil with salt and pepper.

The range of portion sizes can help you meet your specific needs (which depend on age, gender, and activity level). The smaller portions are for women and the larger ones are for men. However, if you find that you are a little hungry on the plan, increase your portion sizes slightly so that you feel satiated.

It's time to savor the flavorful taste of life without added sugar.

SUNDAY

BREAKFAST Oatmeal with Eggs ½–1 cup oatmeal made with water or milk of choice and topped with a dash of cinnamon, 7–15 raisins, and 1 Tbsp almond slivers; served with 1–2 eggs, cooked

LUNCH Turkey Lettuce Wrap Stuff 4–6 oz fresh turkey and 1 oz cheese into lettuce leaf wraps with 2 tsp mayonnaise spread on the lettuce leaves; serve with 1 apple and 1 cup celery sticks and cucumber slices

SNACK ½–1 cup plain yogurt topped with 4 dried cherries and 1 tsp chia seeds or ground flaxseeds

DINNER Lemon Salmon Bake 6–8 oz salmon baked with lemon slices and seasoned with lemon pepper; served with ½–1 cup brown rice cooked in low-sodium chicken broth, ½ cup cooked carrots sprinkled with cinnamon, and 1½–2 cups cooked green beans

MONDAY

BREAKFAST Yogurt Parfait 6–8 oz plain Greek yogurt topped with ¼–½ cup blueberries and 1–1½ Tbsp sunflower seeds

LUNCH Cobb Salad 4 oz fresh turkey, 1 oz cheese, and 2–4 cups greens, dressed in 2 Tbsp balsamic vinaigrette (see page 240); served with 1 orange

SNACK trail mix made with 10 almonds, 1 Tbsp unsweetened coconut flakes, and 1–2 tsp sunflower seeds

DINNER Turkey Meatballs with Pasta 2–4 large ground turkey meatballs and 1 cup whole wheat pasta topped with ½ cup pasta sauce; served with 1–2 cups cooked broccoli and a side salad dressed with 1 Tbsp Italian dressing

TUESDAY

BREAKFAST Avocado Toast with Fried Eggs 1 slice whole-grain toast topped with ¼–½ avocado, smashed; 1–2 fried eggs; tomato slices; and pepper to taste

LUNCH Tuna Salad Pita Sandwich 4–6 oz canned tuna, 2 Tbsp mayonnaise, and 2 Tbsp chopped celery served in a whole wheat pita with 2 lettuce leaves; and 12 baby carrots and ½ cucumber, sliced, on the side

SNACK 1 oz cheese and an apple

DINNER Salmon and Veggie Sauté 6–8 oz roasted salmon served with 2–3 cups sautéed spinach and mushrooms and ½ cup roasted sweet potato chunks on the side

WEDNESDAY

BREAKFAST Veggie Scramble 2 eggs, ½ cup cooked vegetables, dash of hot pepper sauce, and 1 oz cheddar cheese topped with ½ cup black beans

LUNCH Chicken Salad 4–6 oz grilled chicken breast, diced; 1 Tbsp mayonnaise; and 7–15 raisins, serve in 1 red pepper with 1 cup cantaloupe chunks on the side

SNACK 2 celery stalks cut into strips with 1–2 Tbsp nut butter

DINNER Veggie Burger High-protein veggie burger (at least 10 g protein) topped with 1 oz pepper-Jack cheese and 1–2 Tbsp salsa, served on a whole-grain bun with a side salad made with 2–3 cups leafy greens and ½–1 cup salad vegetables tossed with 2 Tbsp extra-virgin olive oil and red wine vinegar; with 1 sliced kiwi on the side

THURSDAY

BREAKFAST Nut Butter–Banana Toast 1–2 slices whole-grain toast, 1–2 Tbsp nut butter, topped with 5–10 thin banana rounds; served with ¼–½ cup plain Greek yogurt and ¼ cup blueberries

LUNCH Turkey & Mozzarella Open-Faced Sandwich 3–6 oz sliced smoked turkey, 1 oz sliced mozzarella cheese, tomato slices, and fresh basil leaves on a slice of whole wheat bread; served with 1 cup sliced cucumbers and ½–1 cup melon

SNACK ¼ cup hummus and ½ cup baby carrots

DINNER Tuna-Kale Whole Wheat Pasta Toss 1 can drained tuna with 1–2 cups sautéed kale, ½ cup diced roasted red pepper, ½ cup whole wheat pasta, and 1–2 Tbsp extra-virgin olive oil, lemon juice, and zest

FRIDAY

BREAKFAST Veggie Scramble 1–2 scrambled eggs served with ½ cup sautéed spinach, mushrooms, and onions; and ½ pink grapefruit topped with 1 Tbsp toasted, chopped nuts on the side

LUNCH Poke Bowl 4–6 oz smoked wild salmon served over 1 cup cooked riced cauliflower, ½ cup cooked brown rice; ½ cucumber, chopped; and ¼–½ avocado; served with 1 clementine on the side

SNACK ½ cup salsa, ¼ cup guacamole, and ½ large cucumber, sliced

DINNER Grilled Pork Chop & Portobello 4–6 oz grilled lean pork chop topped with mustard, pepper, and 1 grilled large portobello mushroom; served with ½ cup grilled eggplant or zucchini, cooled and diced and served over 1 cup whole wheat couscous

SATURDAY

BREAKFAST Cottage Cheese with Strawberries ½–1 cup cottage cheese topped with 1–2 tsp chia seeds or ground flaxseeds and ½–1 cup sliced strawberries

LUNCH Grilled Chicken & Portobello Salad 4–6 oz grilled chicken; 1 oz blue cheese; 1–2 large grilled portobello mushrooms, sliced; served on a bed of 2–4 cups endive and arugula dressed in 2 Tbsp olive oil and balsamic vinegar

SNACK 100-calorie microwaveable popcorn bag, lightly buttered

DINNER Shrimp Stir-Fry with Brown Rice 10–15 jumbo shrimp sautéed in 1–2 Tbsp canola or avocado oil with ½–1 cup sliced mushrooms, snap peas, sliced red bell pepper, and 1–2 Tbsp lower-sodium soy sauce; served with 1 cup cooked brown rice mixed with ½ cup cooked riced cauliflower

DESSERT (OPTIONAL) 1 apple sliced in half and topped with a dash of cinnamon, baked until tender

Symptoms from added sugar withdrawal may include anxiety or restlessness and may last for a few days. In the meantime, fresh fruit, and other ingredients that punch up the flavor such as toasted nuts, unsweetened coconut, and cinnamon can help you cope.

WEEK TWO

SUNDAY

BREAKFAST French Toast
1–2 slices French toast made
with 1–2 slices whole wheat
bread, 1 beaten egg, and a
dash of cinnamon, topped with
¼–½ cup part-skim ricotta or
cottage cheese and ½ cup
sliced strawberries

**LUNCH Chicken & Broccoli
Rabe with Pear Salad** 4–6 oz
grilled chicken breast, 1–2 cups
broccoli rabe sautéed with
garlic and 1 Tbsp extra-virgin
olive oil, served with 1–2 cups
mixed greens, ½ pear, sliced,
1 oz goat cheese, and 1 Tbsp
salad dressing

SNACK ¼ cup pistachios
served with ¼–½ cup berries

DINNER Beef Burrito Bowl
4–6 oz sautéed lean ground beef
and ½ cup black beans served
over 2 cups shredded lettuce,
topped with diced tomato, 1 oz
shredded mozzarella cheese, and
¼ –⅓ cup guacamole; served
with ¼–½ cup cubed melon

MONDAY

**BREAKFAST Cottage Cheese
& Cantaloupe** ½–1 cup cottage
cheese topped with ½–1 cup
cantaloupe chunks; served with
1–2 Tbsp slivered or chopped nuts

LUNCH Italian Sandwich Melt
1 oz mozzarella cheese over
1 slice whole-wheat bread
layered with 3–4 oz sliced
prosciutto and fresh basil leaves;
served with 5 sliced black olives
tossed with 1 cup marinated
mushrooms and artichokes and
1 orange on the side

SNACK ¼ cup hummus and
1 cup cucumber-tomato salad

**DINNER Grilled Steak & Baked
Potato** 4–6 oz grilled flank
steak, 2 cups sautéed spinach,
mushrooms, and onions; served
with 1 small baked potato with
1 tsp butter and ½ –1 cup
cooked broccoli

TUESDAY

**BREAKFAST English Muffin &
Hard-Boiled Eggs** ½–1 toasted
English muffin brushed with
1–2 pats butter and topped
with tomato slices and 1–2 soft-
or hard-cooked egg, sliced;
served with ½–1 sliced peach

**LUNCH Minestrone Soup
& Grilled Cheese** 1–2 cups
minestrone soup, ½–1 grilled
cheese on whole-grain bread
made with 1 oz cheese and 3–4
oz grilled chicken; served with
1–2 cups romaine lettuce salad
with 1–2 Tbsp Caesar dressing

SNACK ¼ cup pumpkin seeds
and 1 apple

DINNER Turkey Chili made
with 4–6 oz sautéed ground
chili, ½–1 cup green pepper
and onion and 1–2 Tbsp salsa;
served over ½–1 cup brown rice;
with 1–2 cups roasted Brussels
sprouts on the side

WEDNESDAY

**BREAKFAST Avocado Toast
with Fried Eggs** 1 slice whole-
wheat toast topped with
¼–½ avocado, mashed, tomato
slices, and 1–2 fried eggs over
½ cup cooked spinach

LUNCH Turkey Lettuce Wrap
Stuff 4–6 oz fresh turkey and
1 oz cheese into lettuce leaf
wraps with 2 tsp mayonnaise
spread among the lettuce
leaves; served with 1 plum
and 1 cup celery sticks and
cucumber slices

SNACK 1 apple, sliced and
topped with 1–2 Tbsp nut butter

DINNER Italian Fish Bake
6–8 oz baked flounder topped
with ¼ cup diced tomatoes
and Italian seasoning to taste;
served with 1 small baked
potato with 1–2 tsp butter and
2 cups cooked vegetables

THURSDAY

BREAKFAST Nut Butter English Muffin ½–1 English muffin, toasted and topped with 1–2 Tbsp nut butter and ½–1 cup mixed fruit salad served over ¼–½ cup plain Greek yogurt

LUNCH Salmon Salad 4–6 oz canned wild salmon mixed with 1–2 Tbsp mayonnaise and 1 celery stalk, chopped; served over 2 cups chopped romaine tossed with ½ cup red grapes and 1 tsp slivered, toasted nuts

SNACK ¼ cup guacamole and ½ sliced red or orange bell pepper

DINNER Grilled Chicken with Quinoa 4–6 oz grilled chicken seasoned with Italian or Greek seasoning, 2 cups sautéed spinach, 1 cup baked eggplant drizzled with 1 Tbsp extra-virgin olive oil; served with ½–1 cup quinoa

FRIDAY

BREAKFAST Protein Smoothie Blend ¾–1 cup plain Greek yogurt, 1 cup unsweetened vanilla almond milk, 1 cup berries, 1–2 cups baby spinach, 1–2 Tbsp almond butter, and ice

LUNCH Cobb Salad 4–6 oz fresh turkey, ½ oz crumbled blue cheese, 2–4 cup salad greens, ¼–½ avocado, 2 Tbsp balsamic vinaigrette; served with 1 kiwi

SNACK 10–15 olives and ½ cup grape or cherry tomatoes

DINNER Turkey Burger 4–6 oz turkey burger patty on whole-wheat bun or English muffin with 1 Tbsp ketchup and mustard, 1–2 slices tomato, and 2 lettuce leaves; served with ½–1 cup mashed cauliflower and 1 Tbsp butter plus 1–2 cups zucchini noodles tossed with ¼ cup diced sun-dried tomatoes

SATURDAY

BREAKFAST Veggie Omelet 2 eggs, 2 egg whites, and ¼–½ cup sautéed peppers and onions, seasoned with Italian seasoning blend and topped with 5 sliced olives; served with ½ pink grapefruit on the side

LUNCH Shrimp Taco Salad 10–15 jumbo grilled or poached shrimp served over 2 cups shredded lettuce, cherry tomatoes, ½ cup salsa, and ¼ cup guacamole, with 1 oz whole-grain tortilla chips broken on top

SNACK ¾–1 cup plain Greek yogurt with ¼–½ cup mixed berries

DINNER Roast Chicken & Baked Sweet Potato 6–8 oz roasted chicken served with ½–1 small baked sweet potato topped with ½–1 Tbsp butter; and 1–2 cups cooked broccoli and cauliflower mix on the side

DESSERT (OPTIONAL) 1 apple sliced in half, topped with a dash of cinnamon, and baked until tender

---

FRUIT SWAPS

Can't find kiwi? Consider these alternative single servings of fruit instead.

1 apple
1 cup berries
2 clementines
½ grapefruit
½ cup grapes
2 kiwifruit
½ cup mango
1 cup melon
1 orange
1 banana
1 cup cherries
1 pear
1 cup pineapple

SUNDAY

BREAKFAST Curry-Seasoned Scrambled Eggs 1–2 scrambled eggs made with 1 oz cheese and a dash of curry powder; served with ½–1 cup sautéed spinach and 1–2 Tbsp slivered nuts

LUNCH Turkey Burger with Sweet Potato Fries 4–6 oz turkey burger patty on whole-grain bun or English muffin topped with lettuce, tomato, pickles, and ¼ cup sautéed mushrooms and onions; served with 1 Tbsp ketchup, 3 oz sweet potato french fries (about 10–12), and 1 cup cooked broccoli

SNACK ½–1 cup blueberries, strawberries, and raspberries topped with 1 Tbsp chopped nuts

DINNER Shrimp Stir-Fry 10–15 jumbo shrimp sautéed in 1–2 Tbsp canola or avocado oil with 1–2 cup bok choy, 1 cup red pepper slices, snap peas, and an Asian seasoning blend to taste; served over 2 cups cooked shirataki noodles or carrot or zucchini noodles; with 2 clementines on the side

MONDAY

BREAKFAST Oatmeal & Eggs ½–1 cup oatmeal made with water or milk and topped with a dash of cinnamon, 7–15 raisins, ¼ cup Greek yogurt, and 1–2 Tbsp almond slivers; served with 1–2 fried or poached eggs on top or on the side

LUNCH Salmon Salad 4–6 oz canned wild salmon mixed with 1–2 Tbsp extra-virgin olive oil and lemon juice over 2 cups leafy greens; ½ cucumber, sliced; ½ cup cooked green beans; and 5 olives; served with ½–1 cup melon chunks

SNACK trail mix made with 1 Tbsp nuts, 1 Tbsp unsweetened coconut flakes, and 1–2 tsp sunflower seeds

DINNER Sloppy Joes 4–6 oz lean ground beef and ¾–1 cup drained fire-roasted tomatoes, diced; served on a toasted whole wheat bun; with 1–2 cups cooked green beans and 1 pear on the side

TUESDAY

BREAKFAST Scrambled Eggs & English Muffin 1–2 eggs served over 1–2 cups sautéed spinach and ½–1 whole-wheat English muffin spread with ⅓

mashed avocado, topped with tomato and red onion slices

LUNCH Soup & Sandwich 2–4 oz fresh turkey stacked with lettuce and tomato on 1 slice whole-wheat bread spread with 1 tsp mayo; served with ½–1 cup minestrone soup and 1 pear, sliced and dusted with cinnamon

SNACK 1-2 Tbsp nuts mixed with 15 raisins

DINNER Grilled Chicken Couscous 6–8 oz grilled chicken breast served with 2 cups grilled asparagus and cherry tomatoes, 1 Tbsp Parmesan cheese, and ½–¾ cup whole-wheat couscous; served with 1 peach on the side

WEDNESDAY

BREAKFAST Avocado Toast and Cottage Cheese 1 slice whole-wheat toast topped with ¼–½ smashed avocado and ½ cup cottage cheese; served with ½ cup strawberries

LUNCH Turkey Caesar Salad 2–4 cups romaine salad with 4–6 oz fresh turkey, 1 oz hard Parmesan cheese, and 1–2 Tbsp Caesar salad dressing; served with 1 orange

SNACK ¼ cup nuts mixed with 1–2 Tbsp chopped dried cherries

DINNER **Steak with Baked Potato** 4–6 oz grilled flank steak, 2–3 cups sautéed spinach, mushrooms, and onions, and 1 small baked potato with 1 tsp butter; served with ½–1 cup roasted Brussels sprouts

THURSDAY

BREAKFAST **Protein Smoothie** ¾–1 cup plain Greek yogurt, ½ cup unsweetened vanilla almond milk, 1 tsp cacao powder, 1–2 Tbsp creamy peanut butter, ½ ripe banana, and ice. For a thinner smoothie, add more almond milk; for a thicker smoothie, add more ice.

LUNCH **Chicken Sandwich** 1 oz mozzarella, 3–6 oz grilled chicken breast, ¼ cup fresh basil, arugula, and 2–4 tomato slices layered between 2 slices whole-grain bread; served with ½ cup grapes and ½–1 cup edamame pods

SNACK ¼ cup hummus and 6 cucumber sticks

DINNER **Tuna-Kale Whole-Wheat Pasta** Toss 1 can drained tuna with 1–2 cups sautéed kale, ½ cup diced roasted red pepper, ½ cup whole-wheat pasta, and 1–2 Tbsp extra-virgin olive oil, lemon juice, and zest

FRIDAY

BREAKFAST **Cereal with Berries** 1 cup shredded wheat cereal with ½ cup milk, topped with ¼–½ cup blueberries and up to ¼ cup chopped pecans; served with 2 hard-boiled or scrambled egg whites, if desired

LUNCH **Chicken Salad** 4–6 oz grilled chicken breast, diced, mixed with 1 Tbsp mayonnaise and 7–15 raisins; served in 1 red pepper; with 1–2 cups cooked vegetables and 1 cup cantaloupe chunks on the side

SNACK 1–2 Tbsp unsweetened, shredded coconut mixed with 1–2 Tbsp chopped nuts

DINNER **Lemon Cod with Quinoa** 6–8 oz baked cod, topped with ¼ cup grated Parmesan cheese, 1 Tbsp melted butter, and lemon juice to taste; served with 2 cups cooked green beans and ½–1 cup quinoa; with ¼–½ cup mango cubes on the side

SATURDAY

BREAKFAST **Broccoli & Cheese Scramble** 1–2 scrambled eggs, 1 oz cheese, ¼ cup cooked broccoli; served with ½ pink grapefruit topped with ¼ cup toasted nuts

LUNCH **Turkey Lettuce Wraps** 2–3 lettuce roll-ups made with 4–6 oz sliced fresh turkey, ¼–⅓ avocado, and tomato slices; served with 1–1½ cups baby carrots and 1 apple

SNACK 1–2 Tbsp nut butter with 6 celery sticks

DINNER **Burrito Bowl** 4–6 oz grilled chicken served over 2–4 cups chopped romaine, ¼–½ diced tomato, ½ diced red pepper, ¼–⅓ cup guacamole, ¼ cup black beans, ½ cup brown rice, salsa, 1 Tbsp avocado oil, and a squirt of lime juice

DESSERT (OPTIONAL) ½–1 cup raspberries served over ¼ cup part-skim ricotta mixed with vanilla extract

Ready to set yourself up for lasting success? Now it's time to reveal the most shocking sugary foods along with the delicious swaps you'll need to control your sugar intake for good.

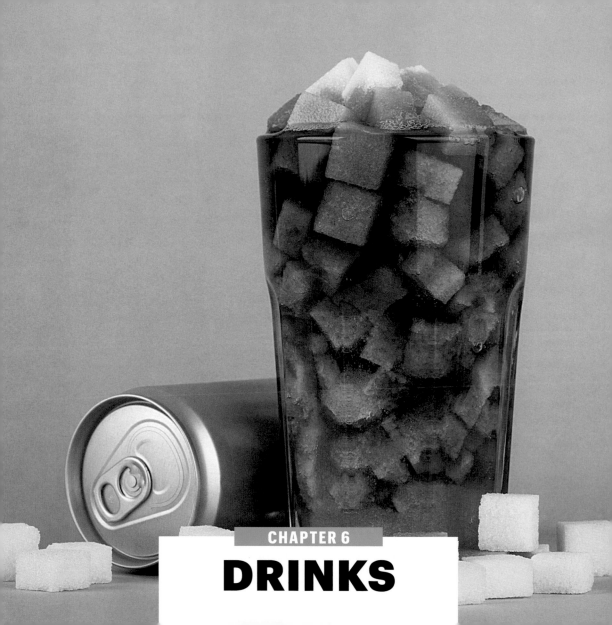

CHAPTER 6

DRINKS

Liquid Dynamite

According to the latest Dietary Guidelines for Americans, sweetened beverages are the leading source of added sugar in our diet, clocking in at a whopping 36 percent of the total added sugar we consume. Plus, in a recent study in the AHA Journal *Circulation*, cardiovascular mortality was found to be 31 percent higher among those who consumed two or more sugar-sweetened drinks a day compared to those who rarely drank them. The chief offenders—soda, energy drinks, fruit punch, and fruit drinks—are essentially liquified sugar that pumps calories into your body without filling you up. The result? We continue to feel hungry, triggering our need to eat and drink more and more.

If that's not a bitter enough pill to swallow, consider this: It's not just soda that's liquid dynamite, but 100 percent fruit juices, smoothies, and even sports drinks that can be serious sugar bombs. With more sugary drinks on the market than ever, you're navigating a minefield of sugar just to quench your thirst. The good news? Here are the swaps and strategies you'll need to enjoy your favorite beverages—and stop drowning in sugar.

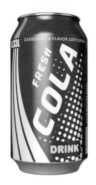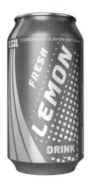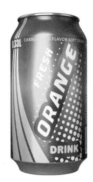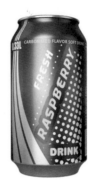

The Facts: The Trouble with Bubbles

It's more than obvious soft drinks are a major no-no—but let's face it, soda can be *sooo* hard to resist. Sweet, fizzy, and with that energizing jolt, it's no wonder soda is just what you need to wash down your lunch, get you through that afternoon slump, or quench your thirst. However, there's hard-core evidence that consuming too much liquid sugar over time can lead to serious illnesses.

FACT Drinking just one 12-ounce can of soda per day can increase your risk of dying from heart disease by nearly one-third according to the *Journal of the American Medical Association*.

FACT People who drink one or two sugar-sweetened beverages per day have a 26 percent higher risk of developing type 2 diabetes compared to people who drink less than one per month per the Harvard School of Public Health. Risks are even higher in kids and teens.

FACT If you drink just one 12-ounce can of soda every day, and do not cut back on calories elsewhere, you could gain up to 15 pounds over three years, says another study from the Harvard School of Public Health.

The Fix: Quit Your Soda Habit!

Even if the science is enough to convince you to stop drinking soda, that's easier said than done. And if you're like millions of Americans who have become addicted to soft drinks, going completely cold turkey is more ideal than real. These fixes can help:

FIX **Count down the cans.** If you drink multiple servings of soda a day, cut back gradually to one a day. After two weeks, switch to three sodas a week.

FIX **Start drinking half soda/half water in your glass.** You'll automatically be drinking less soda as you start hydrating and drinking water. Plus, this will cut back on the sugar, allowing time for your taste buds to change. You won't need that same level of sweet anymore.

FIX **Fill up on water first.** When a soda craving hits, drink a big glass of ice water. You may be reaching for soda automatically because it's so readily available or what you're used to.

FIX **Get your buzz from seltzer.** If it's carbonation you crave, try drinking plain or flavored seltzer water. Buy it by the bottle—or make your own (our pick is the SodaStream machine). If that's not sweet enough for you, add a dash of 100 percent real fruit juice to plain seltzer.

FIX **Try our fixes for 2 to 4 weeks.** This may be easier and more manageable than giving up soda forever. Afterwards, you may not even want to go back to soda—or at least without the frequency you drank it before. Biggest bonus: If you cut back on soda for a while, you'll be shocked at how super sweet it is the next time you pop open a can.

FIX **Make it an indulgence only.** Once you're able to break your soda habit, treat it like any other sugary food—special occasions only. If you love the taste, the occasional can won't hurt.

SODA

Given these outrageous amounts of sugar per 12-ounce can, it's no wonder cola and company are public enemy number one!

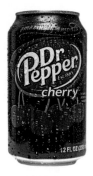 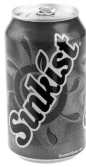 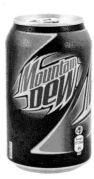 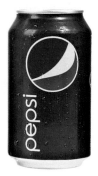 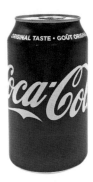

DR PEPPER, CHERRY (12 fl oz)	**SUNKIST ORANGE SODA** (12 fl oz)	**MOUNTAIN DEW** (12 fl oz)	**PEPSI** (12 fl oz)	**COCA-COLA, ORIGINAL** (12 fl oz)
CALORIES 160	**CALORIES** 170	**CALORIES** 170	**CALORIES** 150	**CALORIES** 140
SUGAR 42 g (10½ tsp)	**SUGAR** 43 g (10¾ tsp)	**SUGAR** 46 g (11½ tsp)	**SUGAR** 41 g (10¼ tsp)	**SUGAR** 39 g (9¾ tsp)

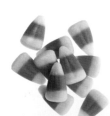

For this amount of sugar, you may as well eat thirty candy corns.

SMART SWAP
SODA

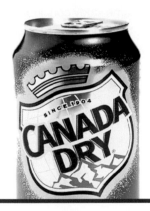
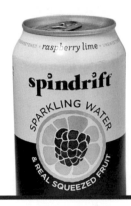

Sugar Shock	→	**Smart Swap**

Sugar Shock
CANADA DRY GINGER ALE
(12 fl oz)

One can only assume ginger is one of the "natural ingredients," but what we do know this bubbly is sweetened with HFCS.

CALORIES 140
SUGAR 35 g (8¾ tsp)

Smart Swap
SPINDRIFT RASPBERRY LIME SPARKLING WATER
(12 fl oz)

Even though this fizzy refresher has both raspberry puree and juice, there's only a touch of added sugar. If you can't find Spindrift at your local market, it can be ordered online from any number of retailers.

CALORIES 9
SUGAR 1 g (¼ tsp)

Sweet Check: Diet Soda

Almost a third of all carbonated drinks sold in the United States are diet. But does that make them a better sweetened beverage?

While the health effects of artificial sweeteners continue to be debated (see, page 42), there's no arguing that a diet version of your favorite soda can eliminate up to 10 teaspoons of sugar (or more). However, there are some serious downsides to diet soda:

• According to research published in *Stroke*, a journal of the American Heart Association, postmenopausal women who drink two or more diet sodas (or other artificially sweetened drinks) a day had a higher risk of stroke and heart disease.

• According to a study in *Trends in Endocrinology & Metabolism*, diet drinks are linked to obesity nearly as much as the sugary ones are. Not a good idea if you're like most people who drink diet sodas to stave off hunger and lose weight.

• This same study concludes that consuming sweet-tasting no- or low-calorie beverages interferes with the body's ability to process natural sugar, which ups your cravings even more.

BOTTOM LINE: Diet soda may be low cal, but any benefit is outweighed by its potential risks. Better bet? Quit your soda habit (see page 93) and say bye-bye to fake stuff.

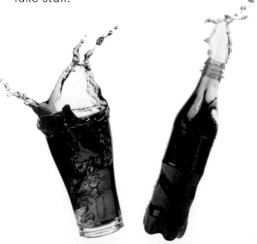

Hello Hydration Heaven!

DIY INFUSED WATER The best replacement for soda, or any sugary beverage, is water—the healthiest thirst quencher. But if you're bored with basic H$_2$O, or you can't wean yourself so easily off sweeter drinks, you can create flavored designer water in a snap.

1 Place 1 to 1½ cups fresh berries, sliced citrus fruit, peaches, nectarines, cucumber, ginger, or diced melon, with or without herb sprigs, in a 32-ounce mason jar.

2 Fill with 2½ to 3 cups filtered or sparkling water. Stir gently.

3 Cover and refrigerate at least 1 hour or up to 2 days.

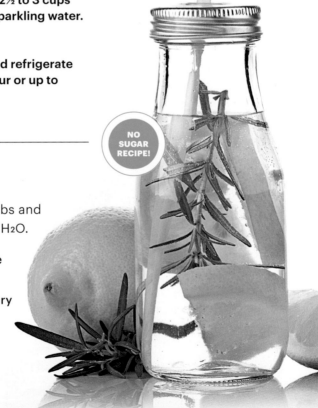

NO SUGAR RECIPE!

Try These Combos!

For a more intense flavor, crush the herbs and the berries in the jar before adding the H$_2$O.

Ginger + Grapefruit + Strawberry + Thyme

Orange + Blackberry + Basil

Nectarine + Lemon + Raspberry + Rosemary

Cucumber + Thyme + Clementine

Lime + Mint + Blueberry + Cantaloupe

Raspberry + Ginger + Mint + Orange

SPORTS DRINKS

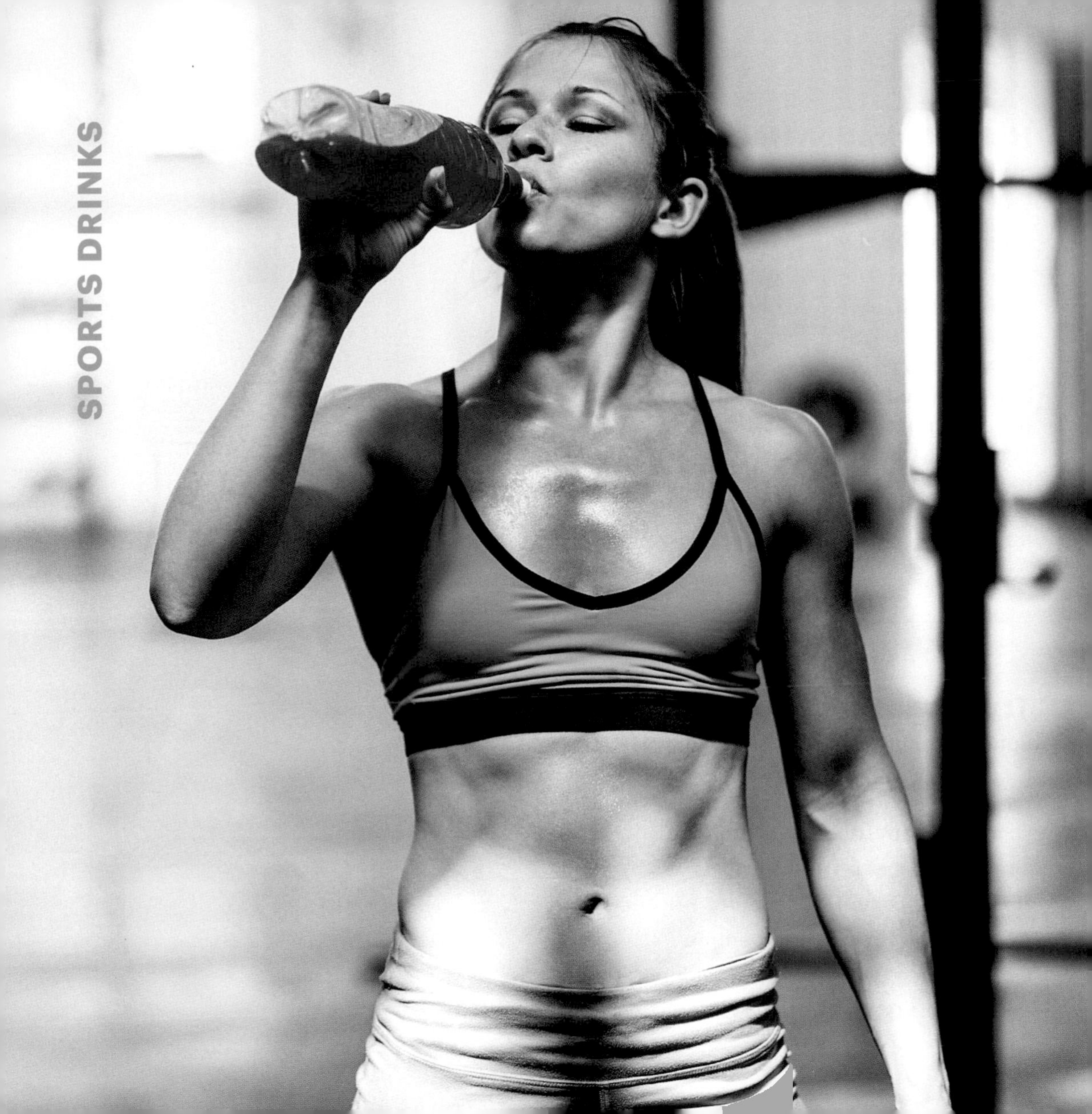

SMART SWAP
SPORTS DRINKS

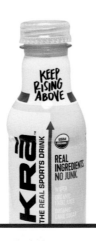

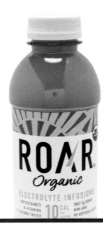

Sugar Shock	→	**Smart Swap**

Sugar Shock
KRĀ LEMON ELECTROLYTE
SPORTS DRINK
(16 fl oz)
Sugar and apple juice concentrate
make this drink far too sweet.
CALORIES 100
SUGAR 22 g (5½ tsp)

Smart Swap
ROAR ORGANIC MANGO
CLEMENTINE
ELECTROLYTE INFUSION
(18 fl oz)
Fruity flavor but with a
fraction of the sugar.
CALORIES 20
SUGAR 4 g (1 tsp)

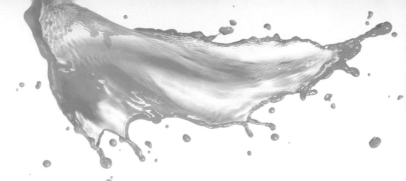

The Facts: Hydrator Hype

With all those cool commercials featuring famous athletes guzzling colorful concoctions, sports drinks are a marketer's dream—and we're buying it. According to the latest statistics, Americans drink over five gallons of the neon stuff per capita per year. Not to be confused with caffeine-boosted energy drinks (like Red Bull or Monster), non-caffeinated sports drinks contain nutrients meant to help you achieve a superior workout while keeping you hydrated. The big sell of sports drinks are electrolytes (sodium, potassium, magnesium) that are added to replace the minerals lost when you sweat. But the carbs in many popular sports drinks are nothing but sugar—okay in extreme cases when you need sustained energy for activities like running a marathon, but less than ideal as your regular workout hydrator.

FACT The most popular brands of sports drinks contain more than double the daily recommended amount of sugar.

FACT According to numerous studies, the added nutrients in sports drinks are effective only during intense exercise lasting over an hour.

FACT According to the University of Illinois Extension, the sugar found in sports drinks delays the absorption of fluids, which slows hydration.

FACT These sugary drinks pack a hearty helping of calories. For casual athletes, that means you're drinking more calories than you're burning.

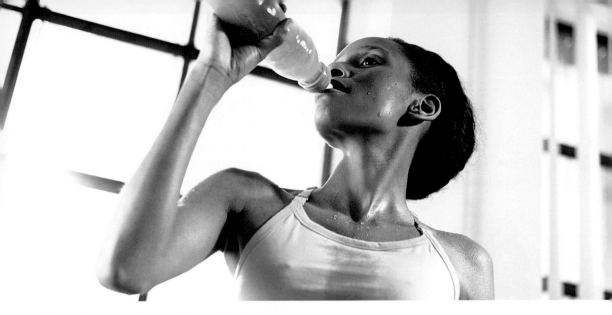

The Fix: Workout Your Drink

You can dilute your favorite sports drink with water to cut the sugar, or get more serious with these simple ideas.

FIX **Try "fitness water" for quick workouts.** Lightly sweetened, or not sweetened at all, these designer waters contain electrolytes plus offer flavor if you're not crazy about plain old water. (Avoid carbonated water, as the bubbles can cause upset stomach.)

FIX **Got milk?** According to a study at McMaster University, low-fat milk is a better option than either a sports drink or water as a source of high-quality protein, carbohydrates, calcium, and electrolytes, especially for kids. (For more about milk, see page 136.)

FIX **Eat these foods.** Avocados, bananas, beans, green leafy vegetables, nuts, and seeds are rich in electrolytes. Nibble those and drink from the tap, and you're good to go before or after you exercise.

SPORTS DRINKS

Don't be tricked by nutrition on the label, as many sports drinks only list the numbers for an eight or twelve ounce serving. That's far less than the whole bottle—which most likely you'll guzzle down while working out.

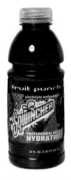
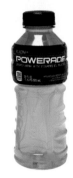
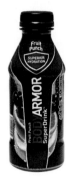
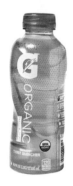
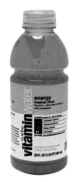

SQWINCHER ORIGINAL, FRUIT PUNCH
(20 fl oz)
CALORIES 175
SUGAR 43 g
(10¾ tsp)

POWERADE, MOUNTAIN BERRY BLAST
(32 fl oz)
CALORIES 200
SUGAR 53 g
(13¼ tsp)

BODYARMOR KNOCKOUT, FRUIT PUNCH
(28 fl oz)
CALORIES 245
SUGAR 53 g
(13¼ tsp)

GATORADE ORGANIC THIRST QUENCHER, PASSIONFRUIT
(16.9 fl oz)
CALORIES 120
SUGAR 29 g
(7¼ tsp)

GLACÉAU VITAMINWATER ENERGY, TROPICAL CITRUS
(20 fl oz)
CALORIES 100
SUGAR 27 g
(6¾ tsp)

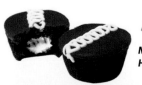

More sugar than two Hostess Cupcakes!

FIVE SUGAR-FREE
SPORTS DRINKS

If you want a fitness water without the sugar
(or calories), check out our five picks:

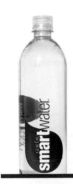 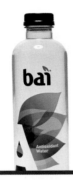 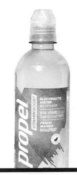 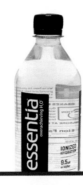 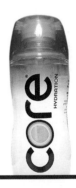

**GLACÉAU
SMART WATER
ANTIOXIDANT**
(25 fl oz)

This top seller
is the smartest
beverage
you can buy
from Coca-Cola.

**BAI
ANTIOXIDANT
WATER**
(33.8 fl oz)

Antioxidants can
help your body
resist the stress
that exercise
puts on cell
membranes.

**PROPEL
PURIFIED
WATER WITH
ELECTROLYTES**
(25.4 fl oz)

Available in
eight fruit
flavors, it's a
good pick if
you're not a fan
of plain water.

**ESSENTIA
OVERACHIEVING
H2O**
(20 fl oz)

A proprietary
process allows
Essentia to create
99.9% pure ionized
water from any
source. It contains
electrolytes too.

**CORE
HYDRATION**
(44 fl oz)

The wide mouth
opening makes
hydrating
quicker, and the
cup cap makes
it easy to share
with friends.

ENERGY DRINKS

While these drinks pack a
power punch, with this much sugar
you're going to crash.

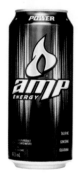

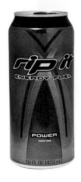

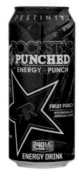

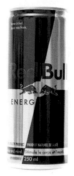

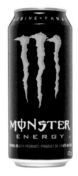

**MOUNTAIN DEW
AMP ENERGY,
ORIGINAL**
(16 fl oz)
CALORIES 220
SUGAR 58 g
(14½ tsp)

RIP IT POWER
(16 fl oz)
CALORIES 200
SUGAR 50 g
(12½ tsp)

**ROCKSTAR
PUNCHED
ENERGY +
PUNCH**
(16 fl oz)
CALORIES 195
SUGAR 60 g
(15 tsp)

RED BULL
(16 fl oz)
CALORIES 212
SUGAR 50 g
(12½ tsp)

**MONSTER
ENERGY**
(16 fl oz)
CALORIES 210
SUGAR 54 g
(13½ tsp)

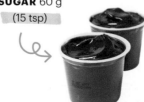

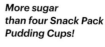

*More sugar
than four Snack Pack
Pudding Cups!*

SMART SWAPS
ENERGY DRINKS

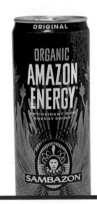 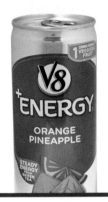 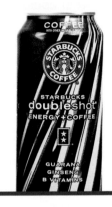 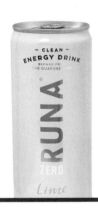

Sugar Shock →	**Smart Swap**	**Sugar Shock** →	**Smart Swap**

Sugar Shock →

SAMBAZON,
ORIGINAL ORGANIC
AMAZON ENERGY
(12 fl oz)

While organic cane syrup sounds healthy, it's just another form of added sugar.

CALORIES 120

SUGAR 29 g (7¼ tsp)

Smart Swap

V8 FUSION ENERGY,
ORANGE PINEAPPLE
(8 fl oz)

Along with its green tea-fueled boost, each can provides one full serving of produce and an entire day's worth of Vitamin C.

CALORIES 50

SUGAR 10 g (2½ tsp)

Sugar Shock →

STARBUCKS
DOUBLESHOT
ENERGY + COFFEE
MOCHA DRINK
(15 fl oz)

Chug this one down and you're over your recommended amount of added sugar for the day.

CALORIES 200

SUGAR 26 g (6½ tsp)

Smart Swap

RUNA CLEAN
ENERGY DRINKS
(12 fl oz)

A trace of organic pear juice concentrate gives this tea-based beverage its hint of fruity sweetness. Choose from lime, watermelon, or blood orange.

CALORIES 0

SUGAR 0 g (0 tsp)

The Facts: Don't Get Squeezed

We are inundated with the message that fruit juice is healthy. Just two examples: Juice bars are everywhere, and fancy juicing machines have become status symbols. And if fruit is healthy and fruit juice is a fast and convenient way to drink your nutrients, what could possibly be wrong? Unfortunately, when it comes to sugar, a lot.

FACT One medium orange contains about 12 grams of sugar, while one cup of orange juice contains almost twice that amount. If you were eating the fruit, you wouldn't consume nearly this much sugar.

FACT Although juice companies are fair in stating their products contain only natural sugars, fruit and fruit juice are not the same. Eating whole fruit raises your blood sugar levels in a slow and controlled manner, and the fiber promotes fullness. But when fruit is processed for juice, the fiber is filtered out or pulverized, reducing the beneficial satiating effects. Drinking juice raises your blood sugar quickly, and after crashing, you'll soon be hungry again.

FACT Metabolically speaking, juice is much more similar to soda (or candy) than it is to whole fruit. According to a study in the journal *Nutrition*, the average amount of sugar in a liter (33.8 ounces) of fruit juice is 46 grams. Compare that to the average 50 grams of sugar in a liter of soda. Yikes.

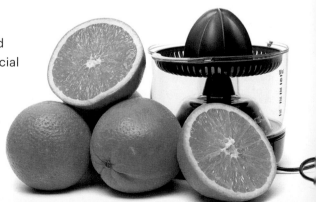

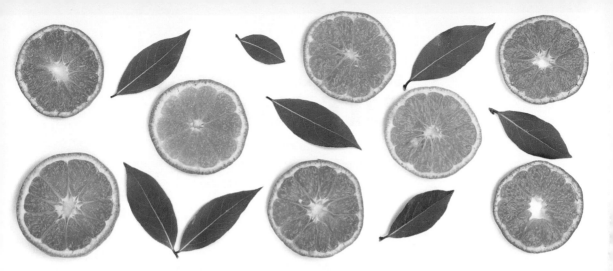

The Fix: Fruit Juice is a Treat

Because 100 percent fruit juice can contain a variety of beneficial vitamins and nutrients, it's not necessary to eliminate it from your diet completely. However, fruit juice should never be considered a substitute for whole fruit. The bottom line: While 100 percent fruit juice is a healthier option than other sugary drinks, avoid the common trap of thinking of it as a freebie. You can't drink as much as you like. But if you keep tabs on the amount you drink, it's totally legit as an occasional treat.

FIX **Try portion control.** Drink juice from a one-ounce shot glass, then follow with a glass of water. Or swap a glass of juice for a piece of fruit and a glass of water.

FIX **Cut your dose.** In a tall glass, add lots of ice, plus 3–4 parts water or seltzer to one part fruit juice. Kids should have no more than half a cup of fruit juice per day.

FIX **Buy green juice.** That is, fruit juice blends with veggies like spinach, cucumber, or celery. Vegetables are typically lower in sugar and calories than fruits. Be sure to read labels to check for added sugars or buy freshly squeezed variations.

SUGAR HALL OF SHAME
FRUIT JUICES

With sugar numbers
like these, you may need to treat
these juices like dessert.

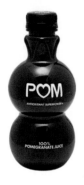
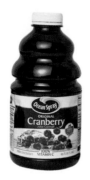
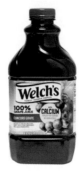
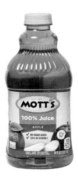
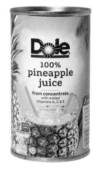

**POM 100%
POMEGRANATE
JUICE**
(8 fl oz)
CALORIES 150
SUGAR 32 g
(8 tsp)

**OCEAN SPRAY
100%
CRANBERRY
JUICE**
(8 fl oz)
CALORIES 110
SUGAR 28 g
(7 tsp)

**WELCH'S 100%
GRAPE JUICE**
(8 fl oz)
CALORIES 140
SUGAR 36 g
(9 tsp)

**MOTT'S 100%
ORIGINAL
APPLE JUICE**
(8 fl oz)
CALORIES 120
SUGAR 28 g
(7 tsp)

**DOLE 100%
PINEAPPLE
JUICE**
(8 fl oz)
CALORIES 130
SUGAR 30 g
(7½ tsp)

*As much sugar as
three Creamsicle
Orange Cream Bars!*

SMART SWAP
FRUIT JUICE

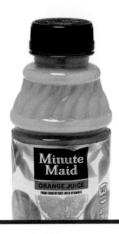 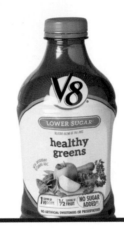

Sugar Shock	→	**Smart Swap**

Sugar Shock
MINUTE MAID 100%
ORANGE JUICE
(8 fl oz)

That's twice the amount of sugar as in a medium orange!

CALORIES 110
SUGAR 24 g (6 tsp)

→

Smart Swap
V8 HEALTHY GREENS FRUIT & VEGETABLE BLEND
(8 fl oz)

Just a touch of pineapple and apple juice sweetens V8's classic vegetable blend without creating a sugar overload.

CALORIES 60
SUGAR 11 g (2"¾ tsp)

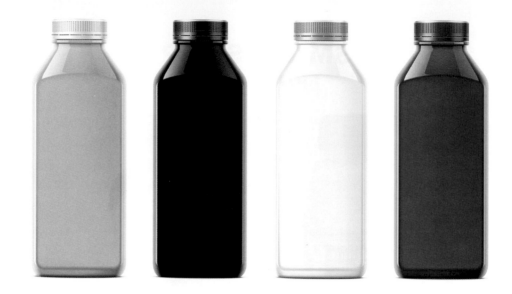

Genie in a Juice Bottle

Buying fruit juice at the supermarket can be a surprisingly complicated task, especially if you want to control your sugar intake. Our Q&A has the answers.

Q: What does "100% juice" mean?

Legally, the definition means everything in the bottle or carton was expressed from a fruit or vegetable. However, it isn't that simple. The juice may not necessarily be from the fruit or vegetable you think you're drinking.

Q: So what fruits are in the bottle?

Fruit juices can be expensive. It's a challenge to manufacture an affordable product when it requires squeezing loads of pricey fruits to produce a single bottle. So companies dilute these products with cheaper juices (e.g., super-sugary white grape, apple, or pear juice). When the label says "100% fruit juice," it may not be the juice from the fruit in the drink's name.

Q: How can you tell what's really in the bottle?

Don't take product name's word for it. Zero in on the ingredient list instead.

DIY Juice!

Talk about a win-win: Making your own juice means you control what goes into it. Follow these tips to craft the healthiest juice:

USE A BLENDER VERSUS A JUICER. That way you can keep the pulp of the fruit, so oranges and pineapple are less of a sugar bomb and you benefit from the fruit's fiber.

INCLUDE VEGGIES IN THE MIX. Cucumber, celery, spinach, and baby kale are good choices. Pair veggies with a small handful each of two types of fruit, like ½ cup of berries and half a banana.

ADD A SQUEEZE OF LEMON JUICE OR A SPLASH OF CIDER VINEGAR. This will mask the taste of vegetables and make the juice taste sweeter without adding more fruit or sweeteners.

CONSIDER THIS A TREAT. Even if it's DIY juice, if it's made with mostly fruit, you should still limit yourself to a couple of glasses per week.

LOW-SUGAR RECIPE

Watermelon & Cucumber Slushie

Enjoy this refreshing sipper that's sweetened with watermelon.

IN A BLENDER combine 1 lb watermelon cubes, frozen; 1 Persian cucumber or ½ English cucumber, peeled, cut into chunks, and frozen; ¼ cup fresh basil leaves; and 4 tsp lime juice and blend until mixture is smooth, adding a little ice water as necessary.

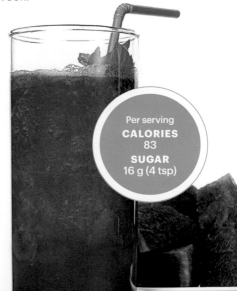

Per serving
CALORIES
83
SUGAR
16 g (4 tsp)

The Facts: Sweet Little Lies

Whether you call them juice drinks, juice beverages, fruit punch, or fruitades, these concoctions have one thing in common: all contain added sugar and have no more than 50 percent real fruit juice. Packaged in brightly colored boxes or pouches, with claims of Vitamin C and antioxidants, fruit drinks are heavily marketed as a healthy beverage for kids and adults alike. But don't be fooled. These supersweet potions are a definite no-no for little ones and for you.

FACT Depending on a child's age and caloric needs, the AHA recommends limiting added sugar to no more than 6 teaspoons (24 grams) per day.

FACT More than half of fruit drinks contain no real juice. Most are 10 percent real juice (or less).

FACT According to a study at Ohio State University, nearly one-third of 2-to 5-year-old kids drink a fruit-flavored beverage each day. In fact, young children in the U.S. consume more added sugar from fruit drinks than from soda, real fruit juice, or low-fat plain milk.

FACT The extra calories and sugar of fruit drinks outweigh the benefits of added vitamins. In fact, Vitamin C deficiency is very uncommon among 2-to 5-year-olds, according to the USDA. On average, young children consume well in excess of the recommended daily amount of Vitamin C. For example, broccoli, bell peppers, and cantaloupe are all good sources of Vitamin C.

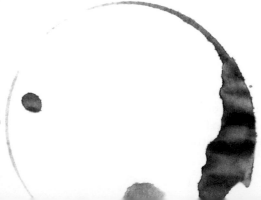

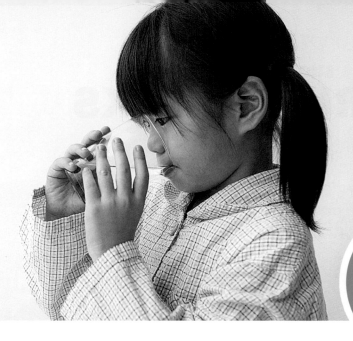

When your child is thirsty, make it a habit to give them plain water first. That ultimate quencher will steer them away from the sweet stuff.

The Fix: H$_2$O for Kids

When kids fill up on fruit drinks, they miss out on that all-important thirst quencher: water. But getting kids to choose water can be a challenge. Here's how to help them drink up and put that juice box aside.

FIX **Make fruit-flavored water.** Mix one tablespoon of 100 percent fruit juice with one cup of water.

FIX **Use frozen fruit instead of ice in ice water.** They'll drink up the water to enjoy the frosty treats. Or freeze berries in ice-cube trays.

FIX **Buy tiny water bottles.** Look for four- or eight-ounce bottles that are easy for kids to hold and drink. Or provide your child with his or her own special drinking cup. Either will make drinking water a special occasion.

SUGAR HALL OF SHAME
FRUIT DRINKS

You won't find much real fruit
juice in these beverages.

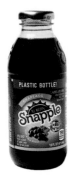

**SNAPPLE
GRAPEADE**
(8 fl oz)
CALORIES 95
SUGAR 23 g
(5¾ tsp)

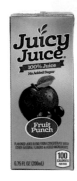

**JUICY JUICE
FRUIT PUNCH**
(6.75 oz)
CALORIES 100
SUGAR 28 g
(7 tsp)

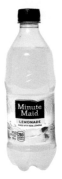

**MINUTE MAID
LEMONADE**
(8 fl oz)
CALORIES 110
SUGAR 28 g
(7 tsp)

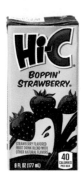

**HI-C BOPPIN'
STRAWBERRY**
(6 fl oz)
CALORIES 40
SUGAR 10 g
(2½ tsp)

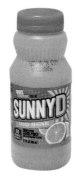

**SUNNYD
TANGY
ORIGINAL
STYLE**
(6.75 fl oz)
CALORIES 50
SUGAR 11 g
(2¾ tsp)

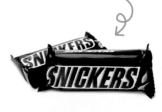

*More sugar
than eight
Snickers Bites!*

SMART SWAP
FRUIT DRINK

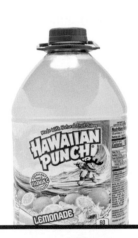
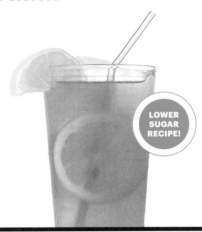

LOWER SUGAR RECIPE!

Sugar Shock
HAWAIIAN PUNCH LEMONADE
(8 fl oz)

What you won't find in the ingredient list is lemon juice—just HFCS.

CALORIES 60
SUGAR 14 g (3½ tsp)

→

Smart Swap
HOMEMADE STRAWBERRY LEMONADE

Unlike Hawaiian Punch, our recipe uses real fruit and naturally sweet strawberries to help slash the added sugar to 9 grams!

Bring 1 cup water to a low boil in a large saucepan over medium heat. Stir in 2 Tbsp honey and remove from heat. Stir in ½ cup fresh lemon juice; ¾ cup fresh strawberries, pureed; and 2 cups cold water. Pour into a pitcher and chill in fridge. Serves 4.

CALORIES 50
SUGAR 11 g (2¾ tsp)

The Facts: Smoothie SOS

Your favorite smoothie can be a super-sneaky source of sugar. Fill your blender with fruit, some fruit juice, a date or two, and a hint of honey, and before you know it, you're chugging down 50-plus grams of sugar. Cue the midmorning sugar crash!

FACT The "tastiest" all-fruit smoothies—those made with fruits high in natural sugar (hello, banana-strawberry with orange juice!) can contain a pound or more of fruit—significantly more than you would ever eat raw. Use fruit juice as a base, and all of that adds up to extra calories and sugar.

FACT Many store-bought smoothies contain added sugar, which increases the calories, not the nutrients.

FACT An average-size smoothie that contains fruit-flavored juices, frozen yogurt, sherbet, sorbet, or ice cream can contain up to half a cup of sugar.

The Fix: A Better Blend

When you make your own smoothie, it's easy to keep tabs on added sugar.

FIX **Rock a new base.** Proper texture is key to a tasty smoothie. Start with an avocado as your texture foundation—it's low in natural sugar and amazingly high in fiber, potassium, and healthy fat.

FIX **Go green.** The healthiest ingredient you can put in your smoothie is a leafy green like kale, spinach, or collard greens. You'll get less sugar by default along with antioxidants, fiber, and other vital nutrients.

FIX **Lose the fruit juice.** Blend your drink with unsweetened green tea or just water, both of which have zero sugar. Or get your protein and calcium with unsweetened yogurt or nondairy alternatives like unsweetened coconut milk, almond milk, or soy milk.

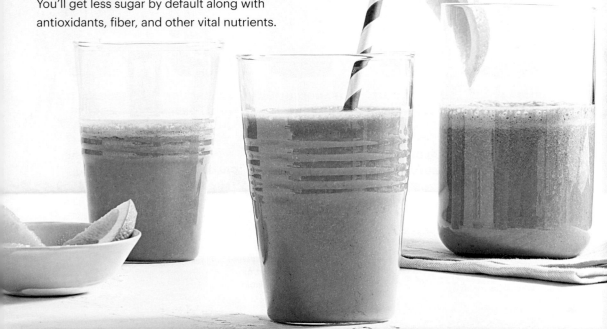

SUGAR HALL OF SHAME
SMOOTHIES

While these smoothies may taste delicious, watch out.
They're often loaded with supersweet juice concentrates
instead of actual fruit, plus added sugar.

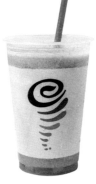

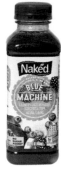

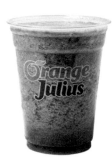

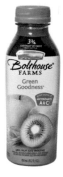

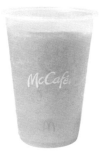

JAMBA JUICE STRAWBERRY SURF RIDER SMOOTHIE
Small (16 fl oz)
CALORIES 250
SUGAR 54 g
(13½ tsp)

NAKED BLUE MACHINE SMOOTHIE
(15.2 fl oz)
CALORIES 320
SUGAR 55 g
(13¾ tsp)

ORANGE JULIUS TRIPLE BERRY SMOOTHIE
Medium (16 fl oz)
CALORIES 370
SUGAR 86 g
(21½ tsp)

BOLTHOUSE FARMS GREEN GOODNESS SMOOTHIE
(15.2 fl oz)
CALORIES 240
SUGAR 50 g
(12½ tsp)

MCDONALD'S MCCAFE MANGO PINEAPPLE SMOOTHIE
Medium (16 fl oz)
CALORIES 250
SUGAR 52 g
(13 tsp)

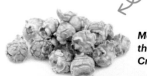

*More sugar than
three cups of
Cracker Jack!*

SMART SWAPS
SMOOTHIES

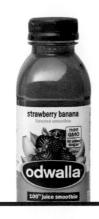
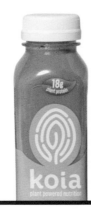
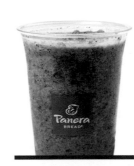
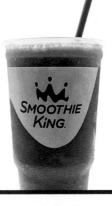

Sugar Shock →
ODWALLA STRAWBERRY-BANANA SMOOTHIE
(15.2 fl oz)

What the name fails to tell you is sugary apple and orange juices are the first two ingredients.

CALORIES 230

SUGAR 47 g (11¾ tsp)

Smart Swap
KOIA PROTEIN CHOCOLATE BANANA
(12 fl oz)

Fruit juice is not the main ingredient in this banana blend. It has the added fiber of chicory root to keep sugar in check.

CALORIES 190

SUGAR 6 g (1½ tsp)

Sugar Shock →
PANERA PEACH & BLUEBERRY SMOOTHIE WITH ALMOND MILK
(16 fl oz)

White grape juice is the main culprit for the sugar load in this drink.

CALORIES 180

SUGAR 39 g (9¾ tsp)

Smart Swap
SMOOTHIE KING LEAN1 STRAWBERRY
(20 fl oz)

This blend of just strawberries, protein powder, and milk is your healthiest option by far.

CALORIES 200

SUGAR 8 g (2 tsp)

The Best Fruits for Your Smoothie

Fruit adds natural sweeteners, but stick to a serving (about 1 cup). And vary your fruit base to ensure you receive an assortment of nutrients. Here are some ideas.

APPLE

This low GI fruit contains 4 grams of fiber—almost 17% of the recommended daily intake.

Natural Sugar: 10 g per medium fruit

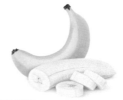

BANANA

A perennial smoothie favorite, bananas can replace the potassium you lose during exercise.

Natural Sugar: 8 g per medium fruit

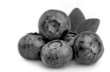

BLUEBERRIES

Blueberries may influence genes that regulate fat-burning and storage, helping reduce cholesterol.

Natural Sugar: 5 g per ½ cup

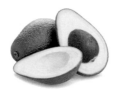

AVOCADO

With barely any sugar, avocados also boast healthy fats to keep you satiated.

Natural Sugar: 1 g per fruit

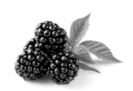

BLACKBERRIES

These berries have one of the highest antioxidant contents per serving of any food.

Natural Sugar: 4 g per ½ cup

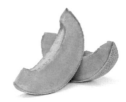

CANTALOUPE

Rich in beta-carotene and potassium to help support your metabolism.

Natural Sugar: 6 g per ½ cup, cubed

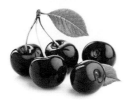

CHERRIES

Cherries contain melatonin, a hormone shown to help reduce jet lag and promote healthy sleep patterns.

Natural Sugar: 6 g per ¼ cup

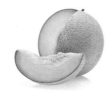

HONEYDEW MELON

A half cup of honeydew provides 17 percent of your daily recommended amount of Vitamin C.

Natural Sugar: 7 g per cup, cubed

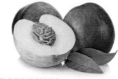

NECTARINES

Nectarines are an excellent source of potassium and a good source of Vitamin A and Vitamin C.

Natural Sugar: 3 g (¾ tsp) per ½ cup, sliced

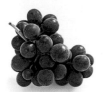

GRAPES

Grapes are high in fiber—plus the red kind is also rich in antioxidents.

Natural Sugar: 8 g per ½ cup

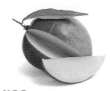

MANGO

This fruit is high in folate which helps support healthy cardiovascular function.

Natural Sugar: 6 g per ¼ cup, sliced

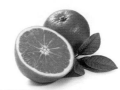

ORANGE

Rich in vitamins, orange sections add sparkling citrus flavor to any smoothie.

Natural Sugar: 8 g per ½ cup, sections

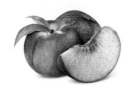

PEACHES

Stone fruits like peaches and nectarines have been shown to ward off obesity-related diseases.

Natural Sugar: 7 g per ½ cup, sliced

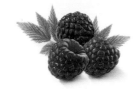

RASPBERRIES

A tried and true smoothie ingredient, raspberries have more fiber than other berries, so they'll help fill you up and keep your blood sugar steady.

Natural Sugar: 3 g per ½ cup

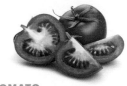

TOMATO

Vitamin A in tomatoes works perfectly to keep your hair shiny and strong. In addition, it also does wonders for your eyes, skin, bones, and teeth.

Natural Sugar: 2 g per ½ cup, diced

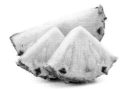

PINEAPPLE

Rich in Vitamin C, manganese, copper, and folate, pineapple can also provide a boost to your immune function and help shorten the duration of colds.

Natural Sugar: 4 g per ½ cup

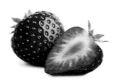

STRAWBERRIES

A mere ½ cup provides more than half your daily recommended amount of Vitamin C.

Natural Sugar: 4 g per ½ cup

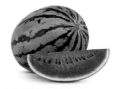

WATERMELON

Watermelon contains Vitamin C and Vitamin B6, both of which help the immune system.

Natural Sugar: 9 g per ½ cup, cubed

Boost It (Without Blowing It)

Kick up your smoothie game with these sugar-free add-ins.

CHIA SEEDS

An excellent source of omega-3s and fiber, chia seeds are also a good source of protein, calcium, iron, and antioxidants. Add 1–2 teaspoons to your next smoothie.

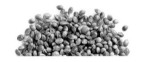

HEMP SEEDS

These little superfoods are a complete protein. They also contain essential fatty acids and a ton of micronutrients to support cellular processes. Grind up to 1 tablespoon per drink.

Smoothies can serve as full meals when they contain a good source of carbs like veggies and fruit, along with protein and fat from milk, nuts, avocado, and/or unsweetened protein powder.

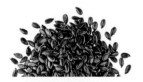

FLAXSEED

This superfood is high in omega-3s for heart health and is an excellent source of soluble fiber. Grind whole seeds first for optimal freshness and use about 1 tablespoon per drink.

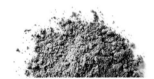

MATCHA

This powdered green tea is made from ground whole leaves. It's known to help assist in weight loss when combined with exercise. A teaspoon is a great addition to green smoothies.

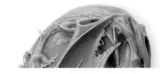

NUT BUTTER

Packed with healthy fats and protein, a few teaspoons of almond or cashew butter will make your fruit-and-veggie drinks taste more like a milkshake, all while leaving you feeling fuller for longer.

The Facts: Specialty Coffee

Coffee boasts some impressive health benefits—it boosts your memory, decreases your risk for diabetes and Parkinson's disease, and even improves exercise endurance—when consumed moderately. But when your cup of joe becomes a speeding vehicle for sugar, it adds a lot of extra calories to what might otherwise be a healthy drink. Supersize it and you're in the sugar danger zone.

FACT Blended coffees contain so much sugar that, consumed regularly, they increase the risk for obesity, the second-biggest cause of cancer after smoking, according to the World Cancer Research Fund.

FACT Indulging in coffee drinks doctored with squirts of vanilla, hazelnut, caramel, or pumpkin spice is pretty much like shooting up pure cane sugar and artificial colors. One ounce (about four pumps) of many flavored syrups contains four teaspoons of sugar.

FACT On average, Americans drink three cups of regular coffee a day. According to the Harvard School of Public Health, it's safe to drink up to six cups of coffee per day. Sweeten each cup with a teaspoon of sugar and you've quickly maxed out on your daily recommended amount.

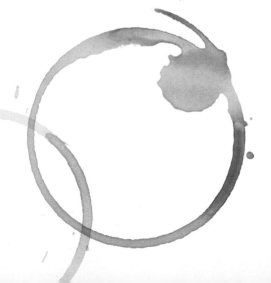

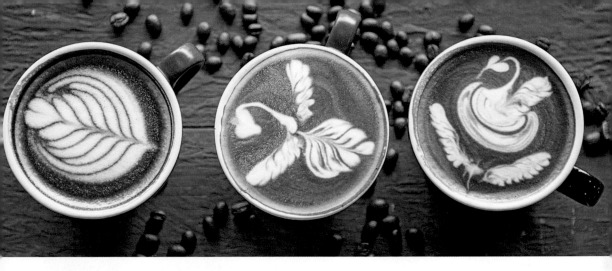

The Fix: A Better Coffee Run

If the idea of black or unsweetened coffee makes you want to gag, or you'd like to enjoy an indulgent java on occasion as a treat, there are a few ways to keep your sugar in check next time you visit the barista.

FIX **Shrink your portion size.** Ordering a small (eight-ounce) drink will slash your sugar intake in half.

FIX **Watch the flavor shots.** Ask for cinnamon powder or unsweetened cocoa instead, or request just one pump of syrup. For a flavor boost without the blood glucose spike, try adding a few drops of vanilla or almond extract to your home brew. They're naturally sugar-free, and chances are you've got some in your pantry already.

FIX **If you typically add sugar to a hot drink, ask for soy milk instead.** Soy milk contains a small amount of natural sugar so you'll still get a touch of added sweetness (and some protein) to help make your coffee more satisfying.

FIX **Don't even consider dessert toppings.** That whipped cream atop your java is supersweet. Ditto for those sugary drizzles, chopped chocolate, or candies.

SUGAR HALL OF SHAME
SPECIALTY COFFEES

Is that coffee or dessert? In the case of these popular drinks loaded with sugar and calories, it's hard to tell.

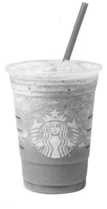

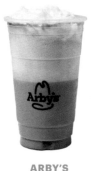

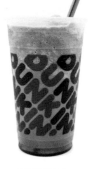

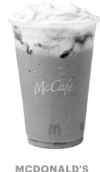

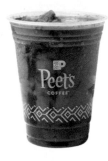

STARBUCKS FRAPPUCCINO BLENDED COFFEE	ARBY'S JAMOCHA SHAKE	DUNKIN' FROZEN COFFEE MOCHA	MCDONALD'S MCCAFÉ CARAMEL FRAPPÉ	PEET'S CHOCOLATE & CARAMEL SWIRL JAVIVA WITH SOY MILK
Grande (16 fl oz)	Small (12 fl oz)	Small (16 fl oz)	Medium (16 fl oz)	Medium (16 fl oz)
CALORIES 240	**CALORIES** 369	**CALORIES** 480	**CALORIES** 510	**CALORIES** 490
SUGAR 50 g	**SUGAR** 68 g	**SUGAR** 96 g	**SUGAR** 67 g	**SUGAR** 77 g
(12½ tsp)	(17 tsp)	(24 tsp)	(16¾ tsp)	(19¼ tsp)

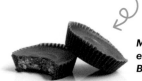

More sugar than eight Reese's Peanut Butter Cups!

SMART SWAP
SPECIALTY COFFEE

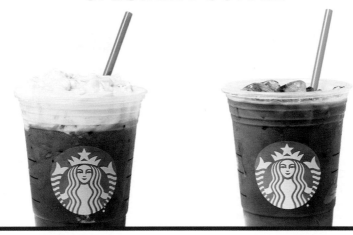

Sugar Shock	→	**Smart Swap**
STARBUCKS ICED CAFFÈ MOCHA GRANDE WITH WHIPPED CREAM		STARBUCKS ICED SKINNY MOCHA GRANDE
(16 fl oz)		(16 fl oz)

Sugar Shock
STARBUCKS ICED CAFFÈ MOCHA
GRANDE WITH WHIPPED CREAM
(16 fl oz)

The trifecta of sugar in the mocha sauce, vanilla syrup–infused espresso, and whipped cream makes this one of Starbucks' sweeter offerings.

CALORIES 350
SUGAR 30 g (7½ tsp)

Smart Swap
STARBUCKS ICED SKINNY
MOCHA GRANDE
(16 fl oz)

Cutting back on the sugar in the mocha sauce, losing the vanilla syrup, and skipping the whipped cream makes this iced brew a more reasonable indulgence.

CALORIES 120
SUGAR 9 g (2¼ tsp)

SMART SWAP
COLD BREW

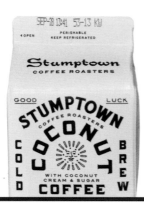

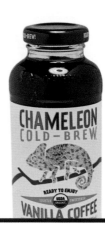

Sugar Shock

**STUMPTOWN COCONUT
COLD-BREW COFFEE**

(16 fl oz)

Coconut cream may make your java dairy-free and vegan, but when paired with the cane sugar in this brew, it's best to take a pass.

CALORIES 300

SUGAR 26 g (6½ tsp)

→

Smart Swap

**CHAMELEON COLD-BREW
VANILLA COFFEE**

(10 fl oz)

Vanilla extract makes it sweet enough. Add a splash of nondairy or fat-free milk and you're good to go.

CALORIES 50

SUGAR 7 g (1¾ tsp)

SUGAR-FREE RECIPE

DIY Cold-Brewed Coffee

There's a reason cold-brewed coffee is a new favorite for many coffee fans. This process reduces the acidity of coffee, which in turn enhances its natural sweetness. That makes it easier to drink without adding sugar. Here's how:

1 **In a small pitcher or 1-quart measuring cup, whisk together ⅓ cup ground coffee and 1⅓ cups cold water until all lumps are gone.**

2 **Cover tightly and refrigerate at least 5 hours or until chilled, but it's best left overnight (not much longer or it will get bitter).**

3 **Strain the coffee through a coffee filter–lined strainer, pushing it through with a spatula. Makes 1 serving (¾ cup).**

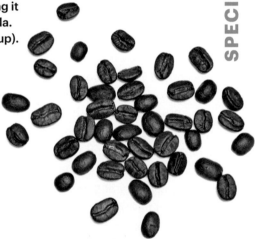

Sugar Bomb: Nondairy Creamers

Look at the fine print and you'll see corn syrup solids and partially hydrogenated vegetable oils topping the ingredient list. Corn syrup equates to sugar and empty calories, while these oils are just a fancy way of saying trans fats—which have been strongly linked to heart disease and diabetes. If you have to go the nondairy route, try sugar-free So Delicious Original Coconut Milk Creamer—its first ingredient is organic coconut milk.

The Facts: Iced Tea and Sugar

America loves iced tea—and not just as a summer refresher. According to a recent report from the Tea Association of the USA, we drank nearly 1.8 billion gallons of ready-to-drink iced tea in one year, making it one of our most popular purchased beverages. Marketers promote the functional health benefits of tea (such as antioxidants, which can improve cardiovascular health and reduce cancer risk). It makes sense that we drink it up as a better-for-you beverage than soda. However, when iced tea is presweetened, it contains a boatload of sugar, throwing any health benefits overboard.

FACT The most popular brands of sweetened iced tea contain as much sugar as a can of soda. Some teas contain more!

FACT Presweetened iced tea can be low in antioxidants because some brands have a higher ratio of water to tea leaves than if you brewed it yourself. Plus, research at the University of Scranton suggests sugar and flavorings that eliminate tea's naturally bitter taste may also dilute its antioxidant content.

FACT Flavored sweetened iced tea can also include artificial flavors and colors.

FACT Terms such as "less sweet" or "a tad sweet" on the label mean it has less sugar than a similar product from the same brand. But that amount of sugar in "less sweet" products can vary from brand to brand. Plus, keep in mind that less-sweet versions can still pack a lot of added sugar.

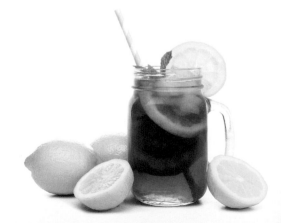

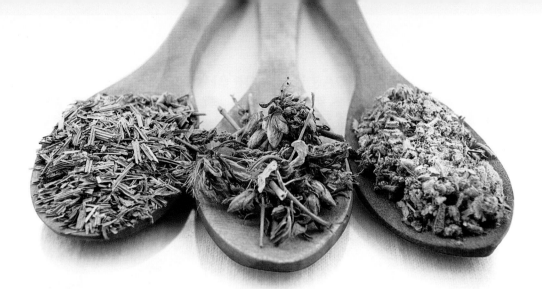

The Fix: "Tea" Up to Unsweetened

On the bright side, there are plenty of unsweetened iced teas on the market. But going from your sweet frosty brew to no sugar at all can be a shock. The good news? It doesn't have to be a bitter pill to swallow with these easy solutions.

FIX **Add a squeeze of lemon.** This should neutralize any bitterness and help you get used to the lack of sweetener.

FIX **Buy herbal iced tea bags or loose herbal tea.** One family-size bag of unsweetened Bigelow Iced Perfect Peach Herbal Tea makes two quarts of iced brew. Plus, herbal tea with fruit flavors is naturally sweet without added sugar.

FIX **If you have to, sweeten it yourself.** Add up to half a teaspoon of sugar, agave, or honey in your glass of unsweetened brew. You'll get some sweetness but with a lot less added sugar than the presweetened stuff.

SWEETENED ICED TEAS

Just call these drinks liquid sugar
with a touch of tea.

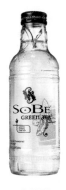 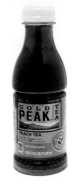 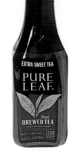 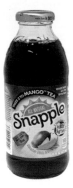 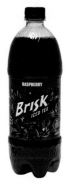

SOBE GREEN TEA (20 fl oz)	**GOLD PEAK PEACH TEA** (18.5 fl oz)	**PURE LEAF, EXTRA SWEET TEA** (18.5 fl oz)	**SNAPPLE TAKES TWO TO MANGO TEA** (16 fl oz)	**BRISK RASPBERRY ICED TEA** (20 fl oz)
CALORIES 200	**CALORIES** 180	**CALORIES** 250	**CALORIES** 160	**CALORIES** 130
SUGAR 51 g	**SUGAR** 45 g	**SUGAR** 65 g	**SUGAR** 38 g	**SUGAR** 33 g
(12¾ tsp)	(11¼ tsp)	(16¼ tsp)	(9½ tsp)	(8¼ tsp)

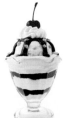

Nearly the same amount of sugar as a Dairy Queen Peanut Buster Parfait!

SMART SWAP
ICED TEA

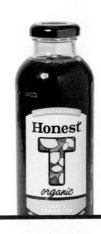 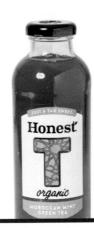

Sugar Shock	→	**Smart Swap**
HONEST TEA, LORI'S LEMON TEA		**HONEST TEA, MOROCCAN MINT GREEN TEA**
(16 fl oz)		(16 fl oz)
As much sugar as a slice of apple pie!		Organic spearmint and peppermint help keep the added sugar in check.
CALORIES 60		**CALORIES** 35
SUGAR 15 g (3¾ tsp)		**SUGAR** 8 g (2 tsp)

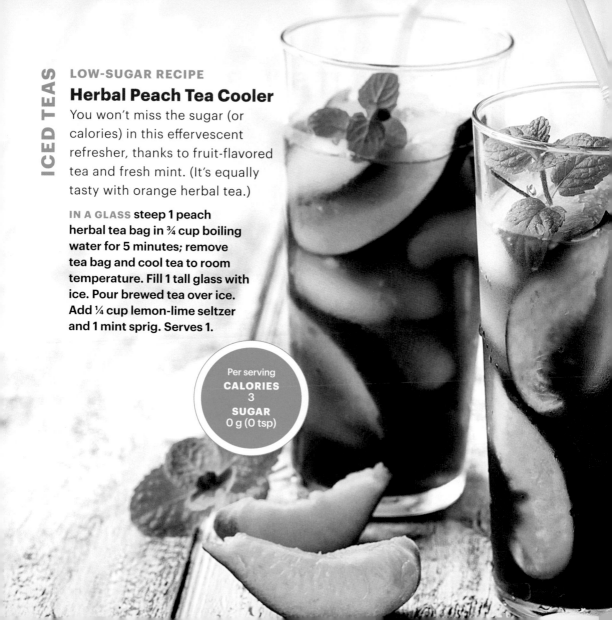

LOW-SUGAR RECIPE

Herbal Peach Tea Cooler

You won't miss the sugar (or calories) in this effervescent refresher, thanks to fruit-flavored tea and fresh mint. (It's equally tasty with orange herbal tea.)

IN A GLASS steep 1 peach herbal tea bag in ¾ cup boiling water for 5 minutes; remove tea bag and cool tea to room temperature. Fill 1 tall glass with ice. Pour brewed tea over ice. Add ¼ cup lemon-lime seltzer and 1 mint sprig. Serves 1.

Per serving
CALORIES
3
SUGAR
0 g (0 tsp)

FIVE SUGAR-FREE
ICED TEAS

Drink up! You won't miss the sugar in these brisk, zero-calorie, ready-to-drink iced teas.

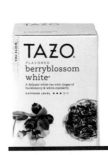 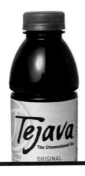 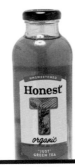 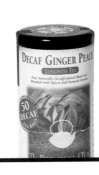 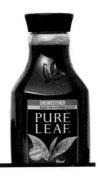

TAZO BERRY BLOSSOM WHITE
(13.8 fl oz)
Made with white tea noted for its subtle, light, and slightly sweet taste.

TEJAVA, UNSWEETENED BLACK TEA
(16.9 fl oz)
Unsweetened black tea can be harsh, but not this soft, smoky brew.

HONEST TEA, JUST GREEN TEA
(16 fl oz)
Vibrant notes of green apple and mango perk up this healthy refresher.

REPUBLIC OF TEA DECAF GINGER PEACH BLACK ICED TEA
(16.9 fl oz)
This decaf tea is enhanced with a tingle of spice and the lushness of peach.

PURE LEAF UNSWEETENED BLACK TEA WITH LEMON
(18.5 fl oz)
Lemony, but not too tart— a plus for unsweetened iced tea.

The Facts: Sugar and Dairy Milk

So what's the real story with sugar and milk? We've got the lowdown.

FACT Regular cow's milk has sugar. However, the sugar in cow's milk comes from naturally occurring lactose, *not added sugar*.

FACT Milk has the same amount of lactose whether it's whole, low-fat, fat-free, or organic milk.

FACT The high protein content (eight grams per cup) slows the body's absorption of lactose, which prevents the risk of sugar highs and lows.

FACT Added sugars in drinks like chocolate milk can double the total sugar of milk (and milk alternatives), undermining milk's healthy benefits.

FACT Flavored powdered milk mixes marketed to kids can contain more than the daily amount of added sugar recommended by the American Heart Association. Malted milk powder adds 14 grams (3½ teaspoons) of sugar, and chocolate and strawberry milk powders add 11 grams (2¾ teaspoons) per one-cup serving of milk.

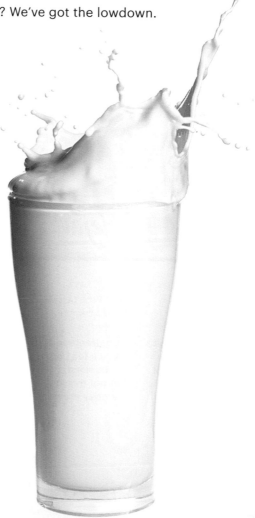

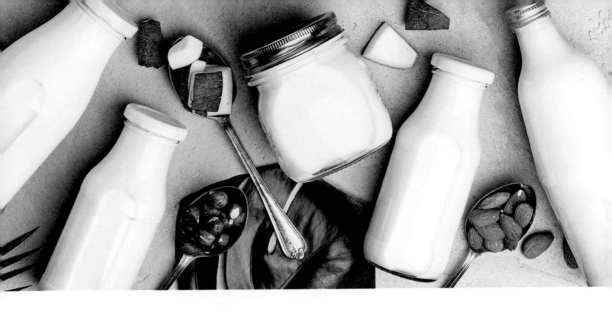

The Fix: Alternative Milks

If you want to avoid lactose, unsweetened alternative milks are a good option. However, there are differences between the varieties.

FIX Unsweetened Soy Milk If you're lactose-free, soy milk is the best nondairy alternative, as it contains the highest amount of protein. The rich body and flavor stand up well to coffee. In general, it can be used cup for cup for dairy milk.

FIX Unsweetened Almond Milk Almond milk, naturally sweet with a nutty taste and a silky texture, is low in calories and chock-full of vitamins and minerals.

FIX Unsweetened Coconut Milk High in saturated fat, unsweetened coconut milk has a creamy consistency and tropical flavor. Use sparingly.

FIX Unsweetened Rice Milk While a valid substitute for people with numerous allergies, this alternative milk lacks nutrients, having only one gram of protein and two percent calcium. Some people find the texture watery and the taste bland.

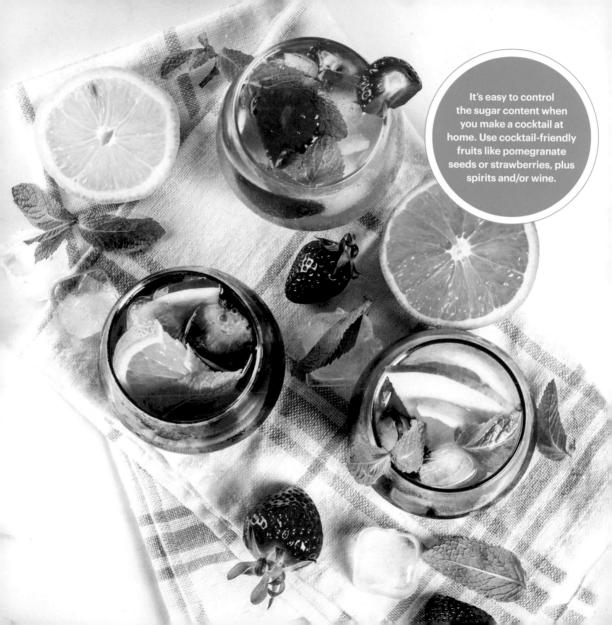

It's easy to control the sugar content when you make a cocktail at home. Use cocktail-friendly fruits like pomegranate seeds or strawberries, plus spirits and/or wine.

How to Order a Less Sugary Cocktail

Use these tips to help you avoid tons of added calories and hangover-inducing sugar.

NIX PREMADE. A 12-ounce frozen margarita has 271 calories and 12 grams (3 teaspoons) of sugar, and a 16-ounce frozen daiquiri has 244 calories and 23 grams (5¾ teaspoons) of the sweet stuff.

CHEERS TO CLEARS. Opt for "clear"—i.e., lower-sugar options—as in wine, champagne, beer, or hard alcohol on the rocks (or with soda) versus creamy drinks.

MAKE IT TOP-SHELF. Choose a premium spirit and sip it slowly on the rocks. You're more likely to nurse your drink over the course of a party rather than throw back sugary cocktails.

AVOID SUGARY ADD-INS. Juice, mixers, energy drinks, tonics, and sugary sodas can dehydrate you and potentially worsen a hangover. Try adding flavored seltzer instead.

ASK THE BARTENDER. Request the fruit or spice flavor in your drink to be fresh. Or order a drink with an alternate mix-in, like herbs or fresh ginger.

SMART SWAPS
COCKTAILS

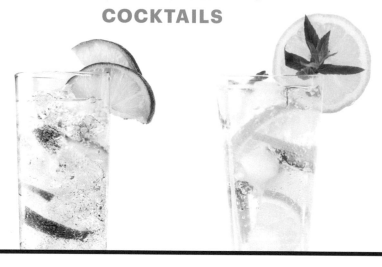

Sugar Shock
GIN AND TONIC

(8 fl oz before ice)

A 12-ounce can of tonic water has a whopping 32 grams (8 tsp) of added sugar. Not a great ingredient for any mixed drink.

CALORIES 207

SUGAR 14 g (3½ tsp)

→

Smart Swap
VODKA AND SODA

(8 fl oz before ice)

Club soda, which is naturally sugar-free, makes this classic cocktail a far better pick.

CALORIES 98

SUGAR 0 g (0 tsp)

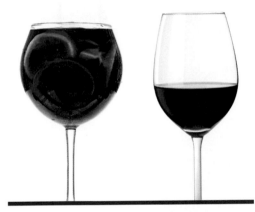

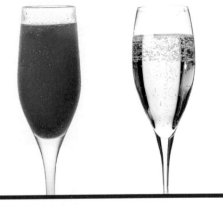

Sugar Shock →
SANGRIA

(8 fl oz before ice)

This combo of red
wine and fresh fruit
may seem like a
good idea, but not
when it's sweetened
with the white stuff.

CALORIES 177

SUGAR 10 g (2½ tsp)

Smart Swap
RED WINE

(5 fl oz)

You're better off
enjoying a glass
of red (or white)
wine solo.

CALORIES 125

SUGAR 1 g (¼ tsp)

Sugar Shock →
BELLINI

(8 fl oz)

This classic duo of
prosecco and
peach puree (cue
in sweet) has
sugar syrup too.

CALORIES 130

SUGAR 9 g (2¼ tsp)

Smart Swap
**CHAMPAGNE
COCKTAIL**

(7 fl oz)

Even though this
cocktail contains a
sugar cube, it's still
less sweet.

CALORIES 192

SUGAR 7 g (1¾ tsp)

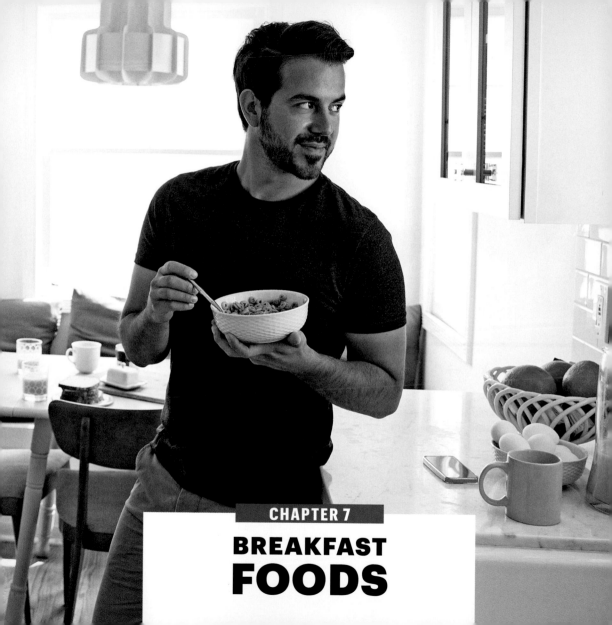

CHAPTER 7

BREAKFAST FOODS

Dessert for Breakfast?!

It's no secret that breakfast is the most important meal of the day. A morning meal balanced in protein, fiber, and perhaps some complex carbs gets your brain and your metabolism going, and it suppresses the hunger hormone in your stomach so you won't overeat at lunch. In fact, the British Dietetic Association recommends that 20 to 25 percent of our daily nutritional requirements should come from our morning meal. But here's the problem: More than 280 million Americans eat cereal for breakfast, and cereal, along with sugary beverages, is among the top sources of added sugar in our diet, according to the Harvard School of Public Health. Plus, quick-fix breakfasts like cereal, frozen pancakes, and breakfast bars may be super convenient for those of us dealing with the busy morning rush to get out of the house, but they can also be super sugary. We'll reveal these and other surprising sugar traps, like granola, along with tasty sugar swaps to help make your breakfast reboot minus the sweet stuff an easy-to-achieve reality.

The Facts: Snap, Crackle... Sugar Rush

Between Tony the Tiger, Count Chocula, Lucky the Leprechaun, and Cap'n Crunch, kids are getting the message loud and clear that sugary cereals are exciting to eat for breakfast. The colorful colors, marshmallows, chocolate, or toy surprises hidden inside the box make it tough to deny your kids (or yourself) those fun foods to jump-start the day. But behind all the jingles and cartoon characters is a major red flag: There's a compelling link between cereals marketed to kids and childhood obesity, a study from the University of Ottawa reveals. Plus, according to the Environmental Working Group (EWG), kids' cereals are even more sugary than they were just a few years ago. Not great news, considering the growing incidence of childhood obesity in America.

FACT Breakfast cereals are the single greatest source of added sugars in the diets of children under the age of eight.

FACT On average, children's cereals contained 40 percent more sugar than adults' cereals.

FACT Almost all children's cereals contained added sugar, according to the EWG, and many contained a third of the amount of sugar a child should be consuming in an entire day.

FACT Kids are not likely to eat just one serving for breakfast. That's because the serving size given on the label does not reflect what Americans actually consume, says the EWG. So kids who eat sweetened cereal every day can wind up with much higher sugar intakes.

For kids ages 2 to 18, the AHA recommends no more than 6 teaspoons (24 grams) of added sugar per day.

The Fix: Cereal Switcheroo

With all the marketing promoting kids' cereals, you may feel you're faced with a choice between buying the extremely sweetened stuff or having your child refuse to eat breakfast at all. But no worries; our fixes are here to help!

FIX **Offer a variety of sweet and less sweet.** Don't go cold turkey. Try purchasing a variety with less sugar and fewer colorants and additives. Start with a ratio of two-thirds healthier cereal and one-third of the sugary stuff, gradually progressing to half and half—or less.

FIX **Let kids control the sweet.** According to the American Academy of Pediatrics, kids will eat lower-sugar cereals when allowed to add a small amount of table sugar and/or fresh fruit to their bowl. In fact, according to the UConn Rudd Center for Food Policy & Obesity, left to their own devices, kids put less sugar on their cereal than manufacturers include in presweetened varieties.

FIX **Switch to ad-free TV.** A recent study at the Dartmouth-Hitchcock Medical Center showed a significant link between TV advertising of high-sugar cereals and an increased intake of these cereals by preschoolers. Going ad-free makes sense when you consider little kids have to hear about sugary treat cereals in order to ask for them.

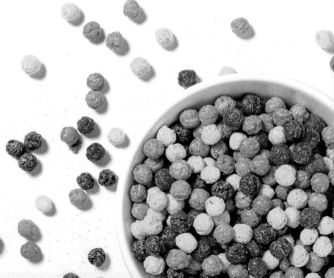

KIDS' CEREALS

Red alert! These cereals contain at least half the daily AHA recommendation of added sugar (3 to 6 teaspoons, or 12 to 24 grams) for little ones—and that's just for one serving. It's no wonder that a child who eats a bowl every day will end up consuming 10 pounds of sugar a year from cereal alone, according to the Environmental Working Group.

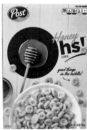 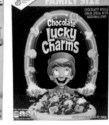 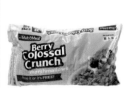 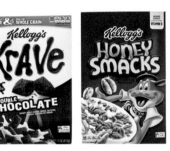

POST HONEY GRAHAM OH'S	**GENERAL MILLS CHOCOLATE LUCKY CHARMS**	**MALT-O-MEAL BERRY COLOSSAL CRUNCH**	**KELLOGG'S KRAVE DOUBLE CHOCOLATE**	**KELLOGG'S HONEY SMACKS**
(¾ cup)	(1 cup)	(1¼ cups)	(1 cup)	(1 cup)
CALORIES 120	**CALORIES** 146	**CALORIES** 160	**CALORIES** 170	**CALORIES** 130
SUGAR 13 g	**SUGAR** 13 g	**SUGAR** 21 g	**SUGAR** 15 g	**SUGAR** 18 g
(3¼ tsp)	(3¼ tsp)	(5¼ tsp)	(3¾ tsp)	(4½ tsp)

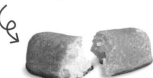

More sugar than a Hostess Twinkie!

SMART SWAP
KIDS' CEREAL

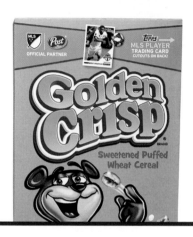 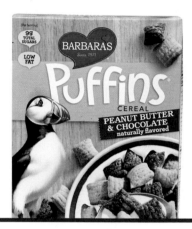

Sugar Shock
POST GOLDEN CRISP
(1 cup)
With Sugar Bear on the box,
Post makes no secret its signature
cereal is extra sweet.
CALORIES 150
SUGAR 21 g (5¼ tsp)

→

Smart Swap
**BARBARA'S BAKERY
PEANUT BUTTER &
CHOCOLATE PUFFINS**
(¾ cup)
A better breakfast pick and real
peanut butter subs in for the typical
amount of added sugar.
CALORIES 120
SUGAR 7 g (1¾ tsp)

SMART SWAPS
KIDS' CEREALS

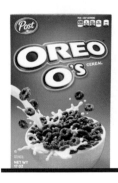
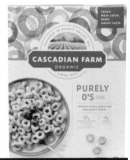
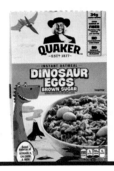
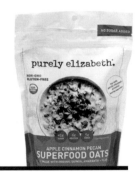

Sugar Shock
POST OREO O'S
(1 cup)

Chocolate O's with a "rich creme coating" means nothing but added sugar.

CALORIES 120
SUGAR 13 g (3¼ tsp)

→

Smart Swap
CASCADIAN FARM PURELY O'S
(1½ cups)

Half the sugar and four times the fiber of Post Oreo O's.

CALORIES 140
SUGAR 1 g (¼ tsp)

Sugar Shock
QUAKER INSTANT OATMEAL DINOSAUR EGGS
(1 packet)

It may have 34 grams of fiber per serving, but the candy negates the health benefits.

CALORIES 190
SUGAR 12 g (3 tsp)

→

Smart Swap
PURELY ELIZABETH CINNAMON APPLE PECAN SUPERFOOD OATS
(⅓ cup)

The only natural sweetener is organic dried apples.

CALORIES 170
SUGAR 2 g (½ tsp)

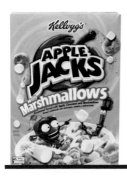 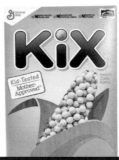 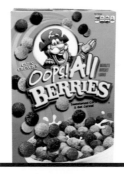 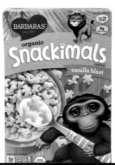

Sugar Shock →	**Smart Swap**
KELLOGG'S APPLE JACKS WITH MARSHMALLOWS (1 cup)	**GENERAL MILLS KIX** (1¼ cups)
When sugar is first on the ingredient list, you know it's a sugar bomb.	Just as crunchy as Apple Jacks (and with more fiber).
CALORIES 110	**CALORIES** 110
SUGAR 13 g (3¼ tsp)	**SUGAR** 3 g (¾ tsp)

Sugar Shock →	**Smart Swap**
QUAKER OATS CAP'N CRUNCH'S OOPS! ALL BERRIES (1 cup)	**BARBARA'S SNACKIMALS VANILLA BLAST** (¾ cup)
Even sweeter than the original. Strawberry juice concentrate is just one of the added sugars.	Lovable character shapes without artificial ingredients.
CALORIES 130	**CALORIES** 110
SUGAR 14 g (3½ tsp)	**SUGAR** 7 g (1¼ tsp)

The Facts: Kid-Sweet for Grown-Ups

Kids aren't the only ones who choose sugary cereal as their morning fuel—adults are sweet on it too. Of the top 10 best-selling cereals in America cited by IRI, a market research firm, only Cheerios is low in sugar, with 1 gram or ¼ teaspoon of added sugar per serving, while our number one sugar shocker, Honey Nut Cheerios, has more than 8 grams, or 2 teaspoons of added sugar per serving. And don't let marketing claims like "Good Source of Fiber" fool you. Even cereals with health claims are often high in added sugar.

FACT Ninety-two percent of cold cereal sold in the U.S. contains added sugar, according to the EWG.

FACT *The Wall Street Journal* reports that cereal manufacturers have increased the sugar content of some cereals after healthier versions failed to win back consumers who were defecting to Greek yogurt and other breakfast foods with higher protein and fewer carbs.

FACT Adults are buying sugary cereal more for themselves—especially millennials, who are eating it as a snack or a dessert, according to Mintel, a consumer research firm.

Turn the cereal box around to look at the nutrition facts before you put it in your cart. A short ingredient list is typically better.

The Fix: Find a Healthy Cereal

Can a cereal be sweetened and healthy? Depending on the type you choose, certain brands can have just as much protein as an egg, the same amount of fiber as oatmeal, and almost as much calcium as a cup of yogurt, once you add low-fat milk. Here are the numbers you need to see on the label the next time you roam the cereal aisle.

FIX **Look for 100 percent whole grain as the first ingredient.** Like whole-grain oats, wheat, corn, buckwheat, or rice. The whole grain should be listed as the first ingredient—not sugar.

FIX **Select brands with at least three grams of fiber (four or five grams is even better) and no more than eight grams of added sugar per serving.** That will be enough to satisfy your sweet tooth without overwhelming your blood glucose levels. The high amount of fiber will slow your body's digestion of the sugars to prevent any energy-draining spikes in blood sugar.

FIX **Avoid any cereal with HFCS or corn syrup (commonly used as cereal sweeteners).** Also be sure there are no artificial flavors, preservatives, or colors.

FIX **Practice portion control.** A cup can be a lot smaller than you'd think, so use a measuring cup to gauge serving size.

FIX **Get a minimum of seven grams of protein for a stand-alone meal.** Scoop out a 250- to 300-calorie serving, or combine it with plain yogurt, milk, fresh fruit, 1 tablespoon of nuts or nut butter, or seeds that are about 100–200 calories per serving.

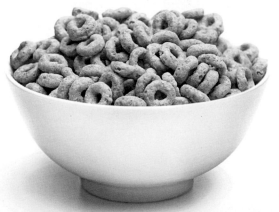

Best Selling—and Too Sweet

Here's a whopper: The average amount of added sugar in America's 10 most popular cereal is a shocking 9 grams (2¼ teaspoons) per serving. (At least Cheerios, the number one seller, is at the bottom of the sugary list).

GENERIC SUPERMARKET BRAND CEREALS
The high sugar content varies by store, so if choosing a store-specific brand be sure to check the label carefully.

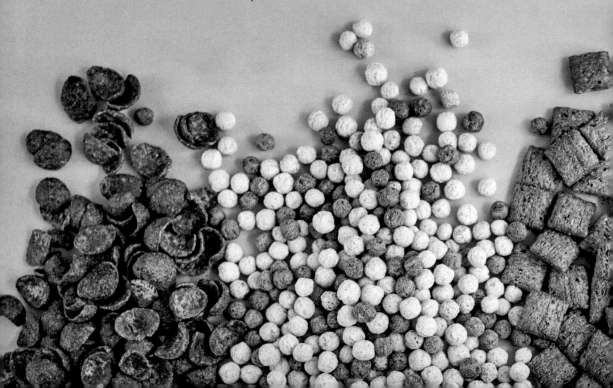

POST RAISIN BRAN
Sugar 20 g (5 tsp)

FROSTED FLAKES
Sugar 14 g (3½ tsp)

FROSTED MINI WHEATS
Sugar 12 g (3 tsp)

LUCKY CHARMS
Sugar 10 g (2½ tsp)

FRUIT LOOPS
Sugar 10 g (2½ tsp)

HONEY NUT CHEERIOS
Sugar 9 g (2¼ tsp)

CINNAMON TOAST CRUNCH
Sugar 9 g (2¼ tsp)

HONEY BUNCHES OF OATS
Sugar 9 g (2¼ tsp)

CHEERIOS
Sugar 1 g (¼ tsp)

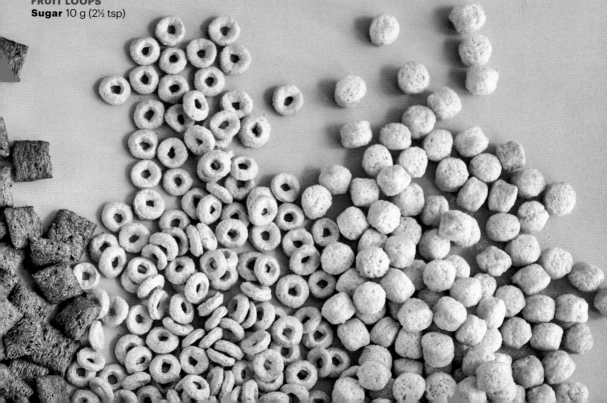

SMART SWAPS
CEREALS

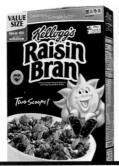
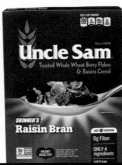
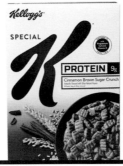
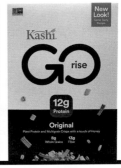

Sugar Shock →
**KELLOGG'S
RAISIN BRAN**
(1¼ cups)

More added
sugar in the box
than raisins!

CALORIES 190
SUGAR 17 g (4"¼ tsp)

Smart Swap
**UNCLE SAM
SKINNER'S
RAISIN BRAN**
(1 cup)

If you can't give
up raisin bran,
Uncle Sam has one
of the lowest amounts
of added sugar.

CALORIES 200
SUGAR 8 g (2 tsp)

Sugar Shock →
**KELLOGG'S SPECIAL
K CINNAMON
BROWN SUGAR
CRUNCH PROTEIN**
(1 cup)

This version of
Special K may
provide 12 grams of
protein, but it's
also twice as sweet
as the original.

CALORIES 160
SUGAR 12 g (3 tsp)

Smart Swap
**KASHI GO
ORIGINAL**
(1¼ cups)

Same amount of
protein as Special K,
but more than
twice the fiber and
less sweet.

CALORIES 180
SUGAR 8 g (2 tsp)

FIVE SUGAR-FREE
CEREALS

Switch to these brands and free yourself
of added sugar this morning.

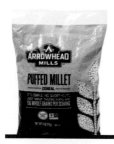 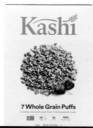 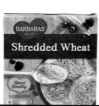 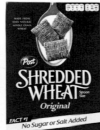 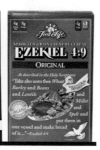

ARROWHEAD MILLS PUFFED MILLET	**KASHI 7 WHOLE GRAIN PUFFS**	**BARBARA'S SHREDDED WHEAT**	**POST ORIGINAL SPOON SIZE SHREDDED WHEAT**	**EZEKIEL 4:9 SPROUTED WHOLE GRAIN CEREAL, ORIGINAL**
(1 cup)	(1 cup)	(2 biscuits)	(1"⅓ cups)	(½ cup)
Because this cereal is so low in calories, consider mixing it with sweetened cereals if you want to reduce your sugar intake.	A tasty mix of hard red wheat, brown rice, oats, barley, triticale, rye, and buckwheat, with a touch of sesame seeds.	Wheatberries are steamed, shredded, and baked for a hearty breakfast.	A hefty six grams each of fiber and protein per serving.	Just as crunchy as Post Grape Nuts, but with eight grams of protein per serving (versus six for Grape Nuts).
CALORIES 60	**CALORIES** 64	**CALORIES** 140	**CALORIES** 210	**CALORIES** 190

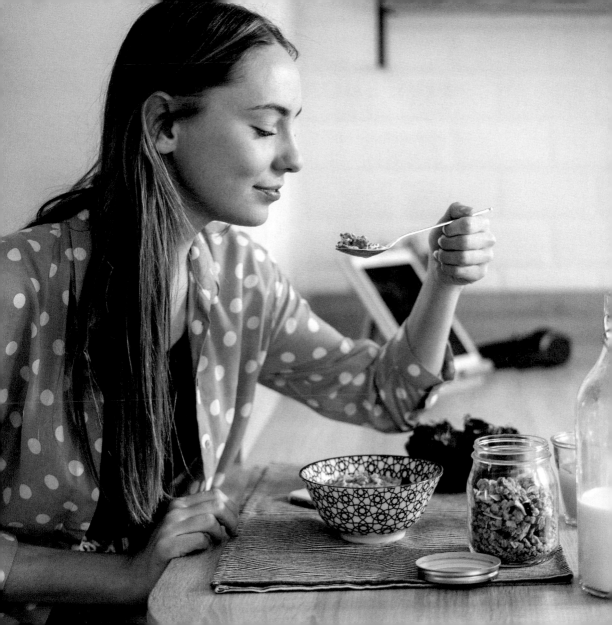

5 Good-for-You Cereal Hacks

These tweaks can make your bowl pack a nutritional punch.

MIX THINGS UP If your go-to cereal is a sugar bomb, you can still enjoy it in moderation. Mix a sweet cereal with a no-sugar-added variety (see page 155) to get the flavor without so many empty calories. Start with ½ cup of each and wean yourself down to ¼ cup sugary cereal plus ¾ cup no-sugar-added cereal.

GO NUTS Peanuts, cashews, and walnuts don't just add a tasty crunch to your cereal—they're also packed with protein. One ounce of nuts has about 5 or 6 grams to start you off on the right foot.

TOP IT OFF Scatter half a cup of berries or sliced fruit over your cereal to get some natural sweetness without added sugar. Fresh fruit also provides fiber and additional vitamins and antioxidants.

HEAT THINGS UP A bowl of no-sugar-added cereal doesn't have to be chilled. To turn plain flakes into a warm treat, heat up a bit less milk than you'd normally use. Spruce it up with a nutritious banana, protein-packed nut butter, cinnamon, and antioxidant-rich unsweetened cocoa powder.

STEER CLEAR OF NUT MILK If you choose rice or almond milk, you'll miss out on a solid serving of protein. Low-fat milk has about four grams of protein per half-cup, but almond and rice milk have less than one gram. If you need a dairy-free option, pick soy milk, which has about the same amount of protein as cow's milk. If you do go with nut or rice milk, add some whole nuts for extra protein.

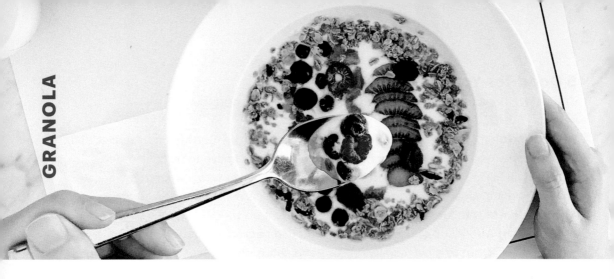

The Facts: Sugar in Disguise — Granola

Granola comes with a giant health halo, being widely marketed as "wholesome" and "natural" and containing whole grains. And while granola can be packed with healthy nutrients, buyer beware—many brands are loaded with copious amounts of added sugar.

FACT The USDA dietary guidelines define granola, along with cookies, cakes, and brownies, as a "grain-based dessert" for its Child and Adult Care Food Program (CACFP).

FACT According to a survey from Morning Consult, a consulting firm, over half of Americans think granola is a healthy cereal.

FACT According to the Center of Science for the Public Interest (CSPI), many brands of granola pack at least 200 calories in each serving, with servings usually listed as a half-cup. But many people eat much more than that in one sitting, which means you could be getting 600 calories or more from one bowl.

The Fix: Make Granola *Grrreat!*

Choose a brand of granola wisely and you can get a bowlful of protein, fiber, and healthy fats without the sugar overload. Better yet, make your own (page 161).

FIX **Know granola is calorie-dense.**
Typically, the recommended serving size is significantly smaller for granola than for other, less dense types of cereal. But that doesn't mean people eat less of it! You'll need to read labels carefully because serving sizes vary significantly from brand to brand, from as little as ¼ cup to ¾ cup.

FIX **Cap your serving at a quarter-cup (no matter what the brand).** Use it as a topping to add crunch to yogurt, fruit, or even pancakes.

FIX **Partner it with lighter cereals.** If you are a granola superfan, mix it with your favorite whole-grain flakes, puffs, or squares, which are less dense.

WHAT'S THE DIFFERENCE BETWEEN GRANOLA AND MUESLI?

Both are made of grains, nuts, seeds, and dried fruit. Muesli is often unbaked and has less added sugar. Granola is baked using a sweetener and oil to bind the ingredients together so they form crunchy clusters.

SMART SWAPS
GRANOLA

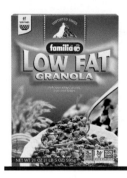
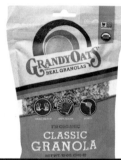
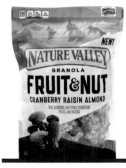
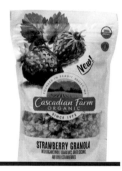

Sugar Shock	→	**Smart Swap**		**Sugar Shock**	→	**Smart Swap**

Sugar Shock
FAMILIA LOW FAT GRANOLA
(⅔ cup)
Don't let "low fat" on the label fool you. These cereals often contain even more sugar than the regular stuff.

CALORIES 210
SUGAR 15 g (3¾ tsp)

→

Smart Swap
GRANDY OATS CLASSIC GRANOLA
(½ cup)
Unsweetened coconut and vanilla extract keep the amount of added sugar under control.

CALORIES 270
SUGAR 6 g (1½ tsp)

Sugar Shock
NATURE VALLEY FRUIT AND NUT GRANOLA
(⅔ cup)
Not only are there three kinds of added sugar, but the dried cranberries are sweetened too.

CALORIES 200
SUGAR 14 g (3½ tsp)

→

Smart Swap
CASCADIAN FARM STRAWBERRY GRANOLA
(⅓ cup)
Organic dried strawberries deliver the same fruit flavor but with far less added sugar.

CALORIES 140
SUGAR 6 g (1½ tsp)

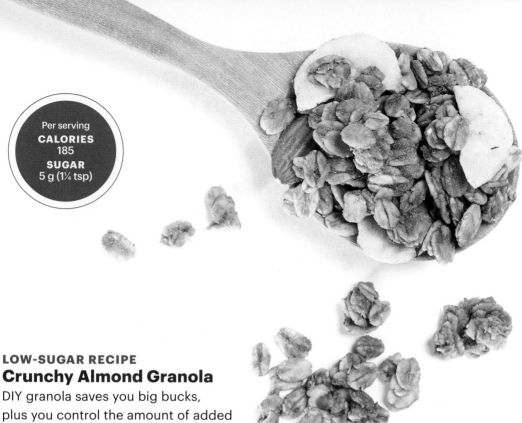

LOW-SUGAR RECIPE
Crunchy Almond Granola

DIY granola saves you big bucks, plus you control the amount of added sugar too.

PREHEAT OVEN TO 350°F. Line 2 rimmed baking sheets with nonstick foil. In a large bowl, whisk ⅓ cup packed brown sugar, ¼ cup canola oil, 2 tsp vanilla, and 1 tsp kosher salt. Add 4 cups old-fashioned oats, 1 cup sliced almonds, and ½ cup sunflower seeds or pepitas (hulled pumpkin seeds) and toss, making sure oats and nuts are well coated. Divide mixture between the prepared pans. Bake, tossing once, until golden brown and crisp, 20 to 25 minutes. Cool completely. Store in an airtight container at room temperature up to 2 weeks. Serves 16.

SMART SWAP
MUESLI CEREAL

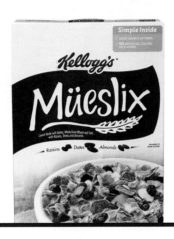 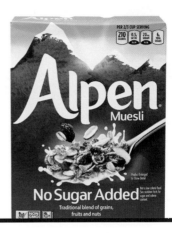

Sugar Shock
KELLOGG'S MÜESLIX CEREAL
(1 cup)

Sugar, dextrose, molasses,
and malt extract are
not what you want to read
in the ingredient list.

CALORIES 250

SUGAR 17 g (4¼ tsp)

→

Smart Swap
**ALPEN NO SUGAR
ADDED MUESLI**
(⅔ cup)

You won't find added sugar,
just raisins in this
blend of oats, wheat flakes,
hazelnuts, and almonds.

CALORIES 210

SUGAR 8 g (2 tsp)

FIVE LOW-SUGAR
MUESLI CEREALS

As fruity and nutty as your favorite granola, but none have more than 1¾ teaspoons of sugar.

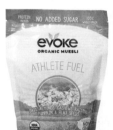 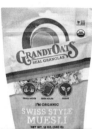 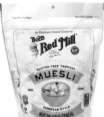 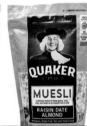 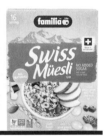

EVOKE ATHLETE FUEL ORGANIC MUESLI
(⅓ cup)

Nuts and seeds provide protein, amino acids, and essential omega-3 fatty acids, with just enough raisins so it tastes great but isn't loaded with sugar.

CALORIES 160
SUGAR 3 g
(¾ tsp)

GRANDY OATS SWISS STYLE MUESLI
(⅓ cup)

Even though it's "loaded with plump dates, raisins, and dried apples," Grandy Oats still manages to keep the sweet in check.

CALORIES 150
SUGAR 3 g
(¾ tsp)

BOB'S RED MILL GLUTEN FREE TROPICAL MUESLI
(¼ cup)

This tropical blend includes dried mango, coconut flakes, and macadamia nuts.

CALORIES 120
SUGAR 4 g
(1 tsp)

QUAKER RAISIN DATE ALMOND MUESLI
(½ cup)

Another brand that contains only natural sugar from the dates and raisins.

CALORIES 210
SUGAR 5 g
(1¼ tsp)

FAMILIA NO SUGAR ADDED SWISS MÜESLI CEREAL
(½ cup)

This classic alpine blend is sweetened with just raisins and dried apple flakes.

CALORIES 220
SUGAR 7 g
(1¾ tsp)

SMART SWAPS
CEREAL BARS

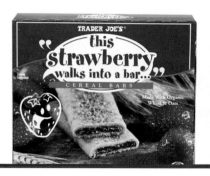 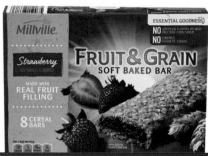

Sugar Shock
**TRADER JOE'S LOWFAT
STRAWBERRY CEREAL BARS**
(1 bar)

With an excessive amount
of added sugar and just one gram
of fiber, TJ's idea of a portable
breakfast falls far short of healthy.

CALORIES 140

SUGAR 17 g (4¼ tsp)

→

Smart Swap
**MILLVILLE FRUIT & GRAIN
CEREAL BARS, STRAWBERRY**
(1 bar)

Eight grams of fiber and less
added sugar makes this chewy bar
a far better way to start the day.

CALORIES 120

SUGAR 11 g (2¾ tsp)

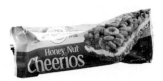

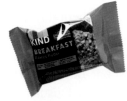

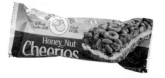

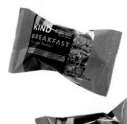

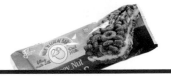

Go for bars that have a real food—a nut, seed, fruit, or whole grain—as the first ingredient.

Sugar Shock
HONEY NUT CHEERIOS
MILK 'N CEREAL BARS
(1 bar)

As if Honey Nut Cheerios weren't sweet enough (see page 152), adding a "milk filling" with HFCS shifts this bar into the candy category.

CALORIES 160
SUGAR 16 g (4 tsp)

→

Smart Swap
KIND PEANUT BUTTER
BREAKFAST BARS
(2 bars)

Thanks to 100 percent whole grains and peanut butter, these bars are rich in fiber and a good source of protein.

CALORIES 230
SUGAR 8 g (2 tsp)

The Facts: In an Instant — from Superfood to Sugar Bomb

A hot bowl of oatmeal, whether prepared with steel-cut or quick oats, will provide you lasting energy to start your day. That's because one cup of plain cooked oatmeal supplies six grams of protein and four grams of fiber—two essential nutrients to keep you feeling full so you won't get hungry midmorning and grab a sugary smoothie or breakfast bar. But the world of oatmeal can get tricky once you opt for instant oatmeal cereals, which usually contain a hefty dose of added sugar.

FACT Instant oatmeal is considered a high-glycemic-index food. The glycemic index (GI) is a rating system that measures how much a carbohydrate-containing food raises your blood sugar levels (see page 22). Rolled oats and steel-cut oats are preferable, as they are considered low-GI foods by the American Diabetes Association.

FACT Steel-cut oats and rolled oats have more iron than instant oatmeal. Instant oatmeal also has slightly less protein because it has been processed more.

FACT Sales of unsweetened boxed oatmeal have declined as much as 25 percent, while dollars have gone up for sugary single-serve oatmeal cups, according to Food Business News, which reports on the food and beverage industry. Targeted at millennial moms, many of these single-serve cereals have the highest amounts of added sugar of all supermarket brands.

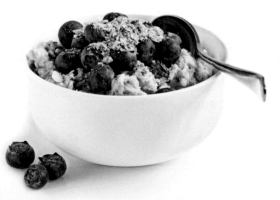

The Fix: Play Dress Up with Plain Oatmeal

You know oatmeal is good for you, but you're not crazy about the taste, so you grab a packet of the flavored stuff or douse your bowl of plain cooked oatmeal with honey or maple syrup. Try these easy fixes instead.

FIX Zap rolled or old-fashioned oats instead of instant for maximum nutritional benefits. Prep rolled oats the same as instant, but microwave them until the liquid is absorbed, about 2½ to 5 minutes. (If you're still all about the instant, look for the plain variety or types that have 50 percent reduced sugar.)

FIX Stick to a half a cup of dry oatmeal and one cup of water, which is one serving size, according to labels. That comes out to 150 calories, leaving about another 150 for your toppings for a filling breakfast that doesn't turn into a sugar bomb.

FIX Avoid sugary stir-ins. Instead of relying on straight-up sweeteners (e.g., maple syrup, brown sugar, or, gasp, chocolate chips), go for alternatives like cinnamon, unsweetened cocoa powder, or vanilla extract.

FIX Choose your toppers wisely. Because dried fruit is so high in natural sugar, it's best to use it sparingly. Consider adding one cup of fresh fruit instead, like berries, sliced banana, or chopped apple. Also add healthy fat and protein in the form of nuts or nut butters, or pour in some milk. The entire bowl should have no more than 7 grams of sugar.

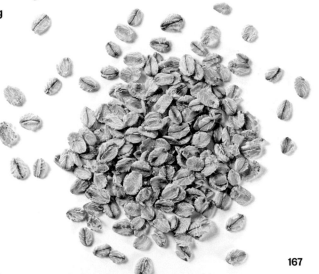

Is Dried Fruit Healthy or a Sugar Trap?

Just like fresh fruit, dried fruit is healthy. But sprinkling too much on top of oatmeal or grazing it by the handful might be too much of a good thing.

Dried fruit is made through the process of dehydration—taking fresh fruit and removing the water. Higher in fiber than fresh and rich in antioxidants, dried fruit makes for a handy and healthy snack. Unfortunately, because fresh fruit contains natural sugars, dehydrating it concentrates that sugar. As a result, dried fruit has a very high calorie and sugar content, including both glucose and fructose.

All fruit has sugar, and the dried and fresh varieties contain almost the same number of calories and sugar per serving. However, a serving of fresh fruit is one cup, while a serving of dried fruit is a quarter-cup. That's a tiny package, making overeating sweet fruits like raisins and dried cherries easy to do. Use these tricks to help avoid that:

• Measure out a quarter-cup and place the fruit in a separate bowl. Don't eat directly out of the package—it's a surefire way to overdo it.

• Limit dried papaya, mangoes, and other fruits that are larger in size and much higher in sugar.

• Enjoy dried fruit with some raw nuts or seeds, or some other healthy fat or protein. That will help reduce the sugar intake and blood sugar spikes.

• When buying dried fruit, look at the ingredient list. The only thing that should be listed is the name of the fruit. Watch out for dried fruits like papaya, pineapple, and tart varieties like cranberries, which contain added sugar.

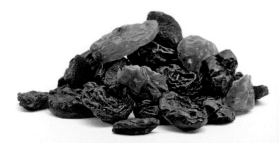

Tiny and Super Sweet

To see how sweet dried fruit can be, check out these percentages of natural sugar content, according to the USDA.

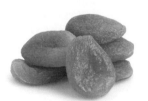

APPLES (1 RING)
Natural Sugar: 4 g
Percentage Sugar: 57%

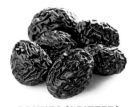

DATES (1 PITTED)
Natural Sugar: 5 g
Percentage Sugar: 64–66%

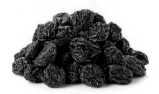

PRUNES (1 PITTED)
Natural Sugar: 3 g
Percentage Sugar: 38%

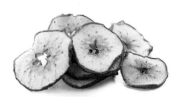

APRICOTS (2 HALVES)
Natural Sugar: 4 g
Percentage Sugar: 53%

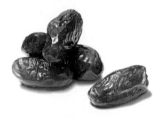

FIGS (1)
Natural Sugar: 4 g
Percentage Sugar: 48%

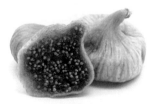

RAISINS (ABOUT 17)
Natural Sugar: 6 g
Percentage Sugar: 59%

HOT CEREALS

Picking up oatmeal at a fast-food chain or casual restaurant might seem like a good thing. If you order it flavored or fancy, though, your supersize bowl becomes chock-full of sugar and additives—knocking this breakfast staple right off its health pedestal.

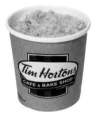 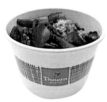 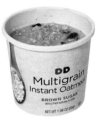 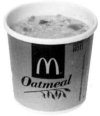 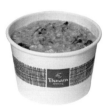

TIM HORTON'S HOMESTYLE OATMEAL MAPLE
(large)
CALORIES 220
SUGAR 20 g
(5 tsp)

PANERA BREAD STEEL CUT OATMEAL, WITH STRAWBERRIES & PECANS
(1 serving)
CALORIES 360
SUGAR 17 g
(4¼ tsp)

DUNKIN' SMART MULTIGRAIN INSTANT OATMEAL
(1 cup)
CALORIES 300
SUGAR 36 g
(9 tsp)

MCDONALD'S FRUIT AND MAPLE OATMEAL
(1 serving)
CALORIES 310
SUGAR 33 g
(8¼ tsp)

PANERA BREAD STEEL CUT OATMEAL WITH APPLE CHIPS & PECANS
(1 serving)
CALORIES 360
SUGAR 18 g
(4½ tsp)

As much sugar as twelve Life Savers candies!

SMART SWAPS
HOT CEREALS

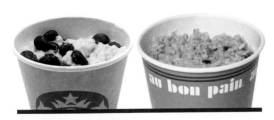

Sugar Shock →	**Smart Swap**	**Sugar Shock** →	**Smart Swap**
STARBUCKS HEARTY BLUEBERRY OATMEAL (1 serving)	**AU BON PAIN SUPERFOOD CRANBERRY ALMOND HOT CEREAL** (small)	**QUAKER REAL MEDLEYS BANANA WALNUT SUPER GRAINS OATMEAL** (1 container)	**BOB'S RED MILL GLUTEN FREE APPLE CINNAMON OATMEAL** (1 container)
This blend of rolled and steel-cut oats may have fresh berries, but it's sweetened with agave (a.k.a. added sugar).	No added sugar makes this three-grain bowl the right choice.	While this oatmeal has five grams of fiber, brown sugar and dried bananas are among the top three ingredients.	Bits of dried apple help reduce the added sugar by half.
CALORIES 220	**CALORIES** 180	**CALORIES** 280	**CALORIES** 270
SUGAR 13 g (3"¼ tsp)	**SUGAR** 3 g (¾ tsp)	**SUGAR** 19 g (4¾ tsp)	**SUGAR** 9 g (2¼ tsp)

The Facts: Sugar Stack

Eaten unadorned, frozen pancakes and waffles may have less added sugar than super-sweetened cereal. But when you slather them with maple syrup or honey, prepare for a sugar spike.

FACT A six-inch homemade pancake has a medium GI value of 67, and a frozen waffle has a high GI value of 76. The glycemic index (GI) is a numerical system from 0 to 100 that measures how much of a rise in circulating blood sugar a carbohydrate triggers—the higher the number, the greater the blood sugar response (see page 22).

FACT Top your pancakes or waffles with just 1 tablespoon of honey and you'll up the added sugar by 17 grams (4¼ teaspoons). One tablespoon of maple syrup or jam will increase the added sugar by 12 grams (3 teaspoons) and 10 grams (2½ teaspoons), respectively.

FACT Five buttermilk pancakes from IHOP has 21 grams (5¼ teaspoons) of added sugar. One plain waffle from Waffle House has 15 grams (3¾ teaspoons) of added sugar. Pour on maple syrup and that's even more added sugar.

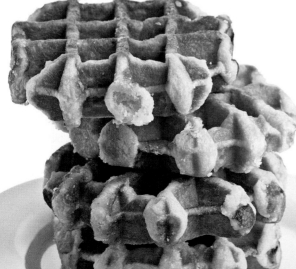

The Fix: A Better Stack

Thanks to these fixes, you can enjoy frozen pancakes and waffles without the sugar load. Better yet, make your own! (See page 175.)

FIX **Scan the label.** Sweeteners like brown sugar, honey, syrup, etc., should be listed toward the bottom of the ingredient list.

FIX **Check the fiber.** This can vary greatly among brands, so look for pancakes and waffles with at least five grams (or more) of fiber per serving. That's the minimum to help slow down the absorption of sugar into your bloodstream.

FIX **Watch out for white (refined) flour.** If there are more than three grams of fiber per serving, chances are your pick of pancakes or waffles will include some whole grains. Check the ingredient list to make sure the whole-grain flour (whole wheat, whole oat flour, brown rice flour, etc.) is listed before the refined flour.

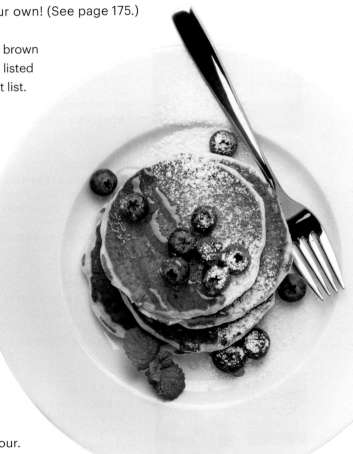

SMART SWAPS
PANCAKES

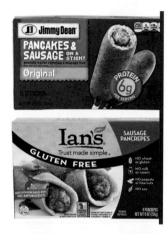

Sugar Shock
JIMMY DEAN FRENCH TOAST PANCAKES AND SAUSAGES ON A STICK (1 piece)
"Cinnamon flavored bits" in the batter does not bode well for a low-sugar breakfast.
CALORIES 230 **SUGAR** 13 g (3¼ tsp)

Smart Swap
IAN'S GLUTEN FREE SAUSAGE PANCREPES (2 pancrepes)
Unlike Jimmy Dean, there's no artificial stuff in the sausage. Plus, the ultra-thin "pancrepes" help slash the added sugar by two-thirds.
CALORIES 220 **SUGAR** 3 g (¾ tsp)

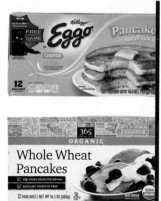

Sugar Shock
KELLOGG'S EGGO BUTTERMILK PANCAKES (3 pancakes)
HFCS and just one gram of fiber per serving make Eggo the wrong move for breakfast.
CALORIES 280 **SUGAR** 12 g (3 tsp)

Smart Swap
365 EVERYDAY VALUE WHOLE WHEAT PANCAKES (3 pancakes)
A hefty five grams of fiber per serving and less added sugar will keep your blood levels stable.
CALORIES 210 **SUGAR** 7 g (1¾ tsp)

No-Syrup Pancakes

Sliced apple baked into these pancakes offers natural sweetness plus pectin, a soluble fiber that may help lower cholesterol.

IN A MEDIUM BOWL whisk 1 cup all-purpose flour, 2 tsp baking powder, ½ tsp cinnamon, and 2 tsp salt. In large bowl, whisk ½ cup low-fat (2%) milk, ½ cup unsweetened applesauce; 2 Tbsp unsalted butter, melted; and 1 large egg. Add dry ingredients and stir just until combined (batter should be slightly lumpy). Peel 1 apple; remove core with apple corer and slice into thin rings.

Lightly coat large skillet with vegetable cooking spray and heat over medium. Spoon ¼-cup scoops of batter into skillet and lightly push 1 apple slice into each scoop of batter. Cook until bubbles appear on sides of pancakes, 1 to 2 minutes. Flip and cook until browned, 1 to 2 minutes more. Transfer to a plate and cover to keep warm. Repeat with remaining batter and apple slices. Serves 4.

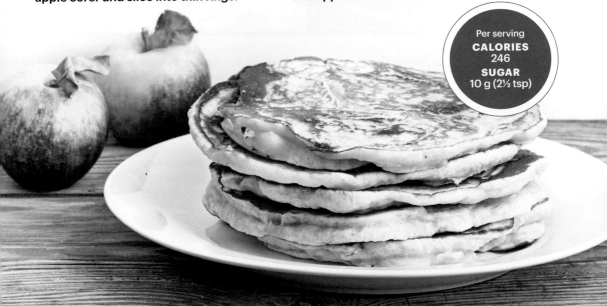

Per serving
CALORIES
246
SUGAR
10 g (2½ tsp)

SMART SWAP
PANCAKE MIX

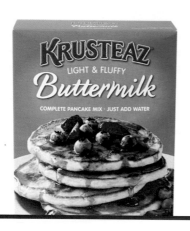 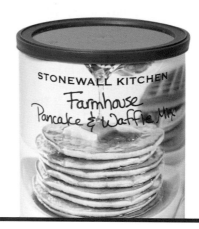

Sugar Shock	→	**Smart Swap**

Sugar Shock
KRUSTEAZ BUTTERMILK
PANCAKE MIX
(½ cup mix)

White flour, sugar, and dextrose are just a few of the health no-no words on this ingredient list.

CALORIES 210
SUGAR 11 g (2¾ tsp)

Smart Swap
STONEWALL KITCHEN
FARMHOUSE PANCAKE
& WAFFLE MIX
(⅓ cup mix)

Unlike most other pancake mixes, this one contains less than 2 percent sugar.

CALORIES 170
SUGAR 1 g (¼ tsp)

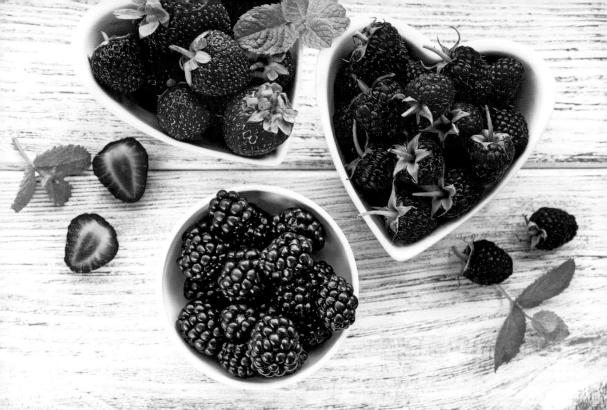

Five Low-Sugar Pancake and Waffle Toppers

Take a tasty pass on the maple syrup—these topper combos
have no added sugar!

Plain Greek yogurt (or crème fraîche) + fresh berries

Diced peaches + chia or pumpkin seeds

Fried egg + diced Canadian bacon

Unsweetened almond, peanut, or cashew butter + sliced banana

Unsweetened coconut milk + diced mango + chopped walnuts

SMART SWAPS
WAFFLES

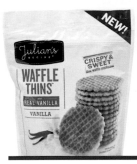
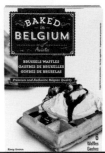
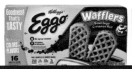
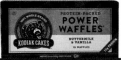

Sugar Shock →
JULIAN'S RECIPE VANILLA BELGIAN PASTRY WAFFLES
(1 waffle)

These waffles feature "pearl" sugar—just another name for larger particles of the white stuff.

CALORIES 250
SUGAR 18 g (4½ tsp)

Smart Swap
AVÍETA BRUSSELS WAFFLES
(1 waffle)

Light in texture with a crisp outer layer, these authentic Belgian waffles deliver the same taste but with a fraction of the sugar. They're available at Trader Joes.

CALORIES 120
SUGAR ½ g (0 tsp)

Sugar Shock →
KELLOGG'S EGGO BROWN SUGAR CINNAMON ROLL WAFFLERS
(4 waffle bars)

Refined flour and table sugar are the first two ingredients in the list.

CALORIES 250
SUGAR 16 g (4 tsp)

Smart Swap
KODIAK CAKES POWER WAFFLES BUTTERMILK & VANILLA
(2 waffles)

Whole-grain flour and a boost of protein powder make these low-sugar waffles a much smarter pick.

CALORIES 260
SUGAR 6 g (1½ tsp)

FIVE LOW-SUGAR
WAFFLES

These tasty picks contain only 1½ teaspoons
added sugar per serving—or less!

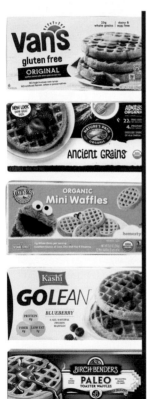

VAN'S ORIGINAL GLUTEN FREE WAFFLES (2 waffles)
Made with whole-grain rice flour and sweetened with just
a touch of fruit juice.
CALORIES 210 **SUGAR** 1 g (½ tsp)

**NATURE'S PATH ANCIENT GRAINS FROZEN
WAFFLES** (2 waffles)
You'll get five grams of fiber per serving thanks to a host
of whole grains like rolled oats, millet, and quinoa.
CALORIES 180 **SUGAR** 2 g (½ tsp)

**EARTH'S BEST ORGANIC MINI HOMESTYLE
WAFFLES** (3 mini waffles)
Perfect for kids, these whole-grain minis are fortified with
iron, zinc, and B vitamins.
CALORIES 60 **SUGAR** 2 g (½ tsp)

KASHI GO LEAN BLUEBERRY WAFFLES (2 waffles)
Naturally sweet, high-fiber blueberries figure significantly in
these waffles. You'll also get nearly half a day's worth of
whole grains—without the artificial colors found in traditional
heat-and-eat brands like Eggo.
CALORIES 130 **SUGAR** 3 g (¾ tsp)

BIRCH BENDERS PALEO TOASTER WAFFLES (2 waffles)
Coconut flour gives these waffles their natural sweetness.
CALORIES 220 **SUGAR** 3 g (¾ tsp)

SMART SWAP
FRENCH TOAST

Sticks are sweeter on average than regular French toast because there's more surface area to soak in the sugary batter.

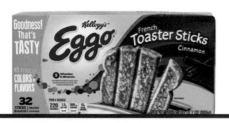
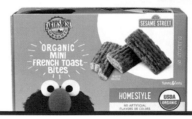

Sugar Shock
KELLOGG'S EGGO CINNAMON FRENCH TOASTER STICKS
(2 slices)

This one contains a trifecta of not-so-healthy ingredients: refined flour, table sugar, and fructose.

CALORIES 220
SUGAR 15 g (3¾ tsp)

$\rightarrow$

Smart Swap
EARTH'S BEST MINI FRENCH TOAST BITES
(2 pieces)

Triple the serving to 6 bites and you still are having less sugar than the Eggos.

CALORIES 60
SUGAR 3 g (¾ tsp)

Healthy French Toast

Just like with our No-Syrup Pancakes, page 175, making your own French toast is the best way to keep sugar in check. All the sugar in this recipe is natural from the berry topping. Be sure to use a whole-wheat bread without added sugar for this recipe. (For great picks, see page 202).

PREHEAT OVEN TO 200°F. In pie plate, whisk 2 large egg whites, 1 large egg, ¾ cup low-fat (2%) milk, ¼ tsp vanilla, and ½ tsp salt. In a 12-inch nonstick skillet, melt 1 tsp butter over medium heat. Dip 8 slices firm whole wheat bread, one at a time, in egg mixture, pressing lightly to coat both sides well. Place 3 or 4 slices in the skillet, cook until lightly browned, 3 to 4 minutes; flip to cook 3 to 4 minutes on second side. Transfer French toast to cookie sheet; keep warm in oven. Repeat with 1 tsp butter, bread slices, and egg mixture. Top each serving with ½ cup berries and ¼ cup plain yogurt for a touch of sweetness. Serves 4.

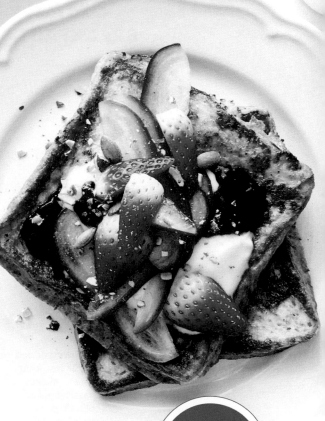

Per serving
CALORIES
280
SUGAR
13 g (3¼ tsp)

SMART SWAPS
BREAKFAST SANDWICHES

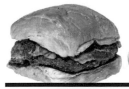
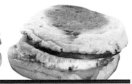
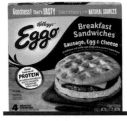
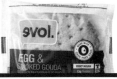

Sugar Shock →
**WENDY'S MAPLE
BACON CHICKEN
CROISSANT**
(1 sandwich)

That's half your
recommended
allowance of added
sugar for the day.

CALORIES 570
SUGAR 13 g (3¼ tsp)

Smart Swap
**MCDONALD'S
EGG MCMUFFIN**
(1 sandwich)

With the lowest added
sugar of all fast-food
breakfasts, Mickey
D's classic delivers
a solid 18 grams
of protein for a filling
sandwich that won't
spike your blood sugar.

CALORIES 300
SUGAR 3 g (¾ tsp)

Sugar Shock →
**KELLOGG'S EGGO
SAUSAGE, EGG &
CHEESE BREAKFAST
SANDWICHES**
(1 sandwich)

Sugar (third in the
ingredient list) plus
brown sugar
and fructose are not
the fixings for
a healthy breakfast.

CALORIES 270
SUGAR 7 g (1¾ tsp)

Smart Swap
**EVOL. EGG
AND SMOKED
GOUDA BREAKFAST
SANDWICH**

This solid protein
sandwich features
whole egg, egg white,
and sweet-and-smoky
Gouda cheese layered
in between two
thin slices of multigrain
artisan bread.

CALORIES 190
SUGAR ½ g (0 tsp)

FIVE LOW-SUGAR
BREAKFAST BURRITOS

Frozen burritos make a fabulous grab-and-go breakfast, especially when they contain no more than one teaspoon (four grams) of sugar.

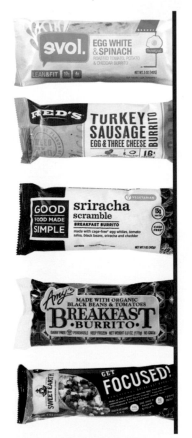

EVOL. EGG WHITE AND SPINACH BURRITO
You'll also find roasted tomatoes and potatoes, Cheddar, and salsa—all rolled in a whole wheat tortilla.
CALORIES 260 **SUGAR** 1 g (¼ tsp)

RED'S TURKEY SAUSAGE, EGG & THREE CHEESE BURRITO
Pepper-Jack, mozzarella, and Cheddar make this burrito extra cheesy.
CALORIES 320 **SUGAR** 1 g (¼ tsp)

GOOD FOOD MADE SIMPLE SRIRACHA SCRAMBLE BREAKFAST BURRITO
Scrambled egg whites, tomato salsa, black beans, cheese, sweet potatoes, spinach, and avocado are spiced up with Thai hot sauce.
CALORIES 315 **SUGAR** 4 g (1 tsp)

AMY'S BREAKFAST BURRITO
Black beans and tofu team up to provide a solid dose of protein and fiber.
CALORIES 270 **SUGAR** 3 g (¾ tsp)

SWEET EARTH GET FOCUSED BREAKFAST BURRITO
This burrito is a yummy mix of scrambled eggs and high-fiber farro, kale, and peas.
CALORIES 310 **SUGAR** 3 g (¾ tsp)

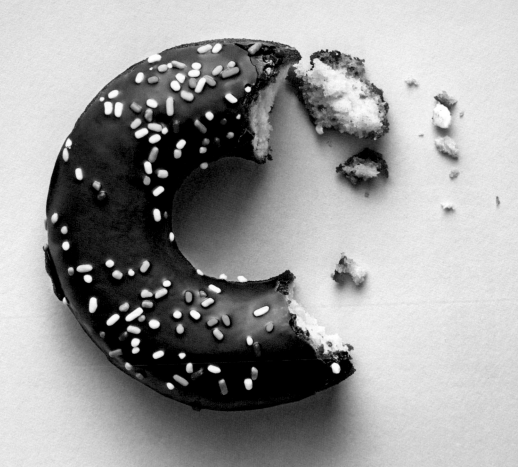

CHAPTER 8

BAKED
GOODS

Baked-In Sugar Traps

If a morning muffin or brown-bag sandwich at lunch is part of your daily routine, there are obvious, and not so obvious, sources of added sugar in your diet. We offer smart swaps for classic baked goods like supersize muffins and also expose the surprising hidden sugar in bakery items like bagels and even whole-grain bread.

The Facts: Muffins

America loves muffins. According to the latest trend report from Packaged Facts, a publisher of market research in the food, beverage, and consumer goods sectors, from 2016 to 2017, muffin sales jumped by nearly 10 percent to $1.17 billion, making it the third-fastest-growing breakfast choice after eggs and drinkable yogurt. Too bad the majority of packaged muffins are so sweet you might as well eat cake.

FACT The portion size of a typical muffin is more than three times larger than the USDA recommendation, according to the National Institutes of Health.

FACT According to a survey from the Harvard School of Public Health, an average coffee shop blueberry muffin has nearly 470 calories, primarily from white flour and sugar. That's nearly double what you'd get from a chocolate frosted donut.

FACT Low-fat muffins often masquerade as a "better for you" choice. However, when the fat is cut back, manufacturers usually add more sugar to retain the moistness and tender texture of a full-fat muffin.

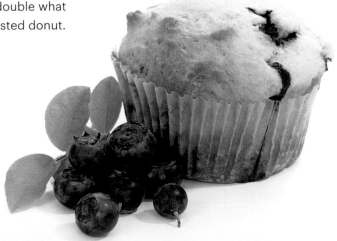

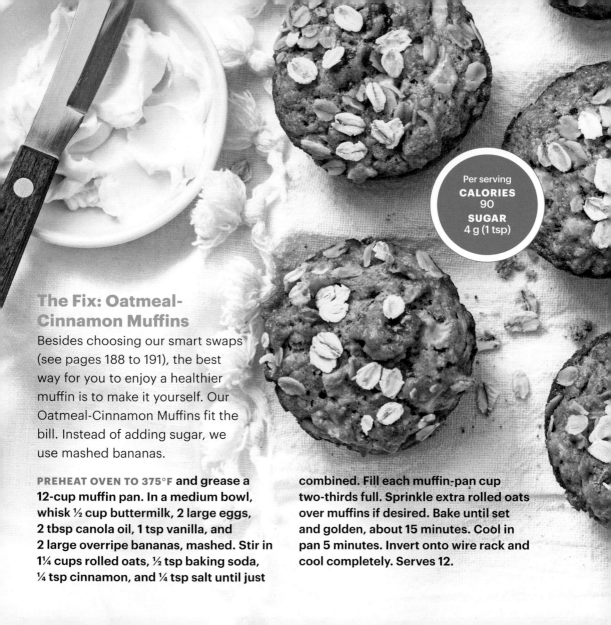

Per serving
CALORIES
90
SUGAR
4 g (1 tsp)

The Fix: Oatmeal-Cinnamon Muffins

Besides choosing our smart swaps (see pages 188 to 191), the best way for you to enjoy a healthier muffin is to make it yourself. Our Oatmeal-Cinnamon Muffins fit the bill. Instead of adding sugar, we use mashed bananas.

PREHEAT OVEN TO 375°F and grease a 12-cup muffin pan. In a medium bowl, whisk ½ cup buttermilk, 2 large eggs, 2 tbsp canola oil, 1 tsp vanilla, and 2 large overripe bananas, mashed. Stir in 1¼ cups rolled oats, ½ tsp baking soda, ¼ tsp cinnamon, and ¼ tsp salt until just combined. Fill each muffin-pan cup two-thirds full. Sprinkle extra rolled oats over muffins if desired. Bake until set and golden, about 15 minutes. Cool in pan 5 minutes. Invert onto wire rack and cool completely. Serves 12.

SUGAR HALL OF SHAME
BAKERY MUFFINS

Visit a coffee bar for your morning cup and chances are you'll encounter the ubiquitous muffin. Dotted with fruit or sprinkled with nuts, muffins may appear to be a better choice than their doughnut neighbors. But when it comes to sugar, these bakery-chain muffins tell a different story.

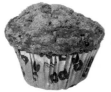

DUNKIN' COFFEE CAKE MUFFIN
(1 muffin)
CALORIES 590
SUGAR 51 g
(12¾ tsp)

PANERA BREAD PUMPKIN MUFFIN
(1 muffin)
CALORIES 580
SUGAR 51 g
(12¾ tsp)

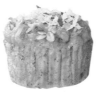

WINCHELL'S PINEAPPLE UPSIDE DOWN MUFFIN
(1 muffin)
CALORIES 510
SUGAR 54 g
(13½ tsp)

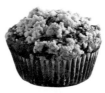

CARIBOU COFFEE FRENCH TOAST MUFFIN
(1 muffin)
CALORIES 490
SUGAR 50 g
(12"½ tsp)

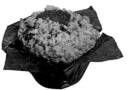

EINSTEIN BROS CINNAMON CHIP MUFFIN
(1 muffin)
CALORIES 500
SUGAR 47 g
(11¾ tsp)

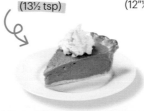

As much sugar as two slices of pumpkin pie!

SMART SWAP
BAKERY MUFFINS

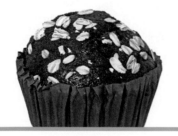
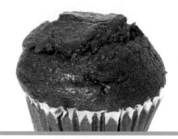

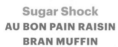

Sugar Shock	→	Smart Swap
AU BON PAIN RAISIN BRAN MUFFIN		**PEET'S COFFEE & TEA BRAN CRANBERRY APPLE MUFFIN**
(1 muffin)		(1 muffin)
This "healthy muffin" has more sugar than a Little Debbie fudge brownie.		This muffin from Peet's is one of the lowest in added sugar.
CALORIES 430		**CALORIES** 486
SUGAR 31 g (7¾ tsp)		**SUGAR** 18 g (4½ tsp)

SMART SWAP
MUFFINS

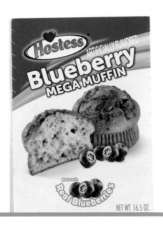 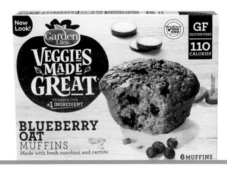

Sugar Shock	→	**Smart Swap**
HOSTESS BLUEBERRY MEGA MUFFIN		**GARDEN LITES BLUEBERRY OAT MUFFINS**
(1 muffin)		(1 muffin)
While smaller than a supersize coffeehouse muffin, this supermarket brand is still a sugar bomb.		Zucchini is the first ingredient in these healthful muffins that have a fraction of the sugar.
CALORIES 560		**CALORIES** 110
SUGAR 30 g (7½ tsp)		**SUGAR** 10 g (2½ tsp)

FIVE LESS-SUGARY
MUFFINS

Don't have time to make our Oatmeal-Cinnamon Muffins (page 187)?
Check out these low-sugar muffin mixes for a tasty yet healthy alternative.

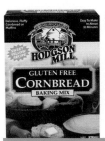 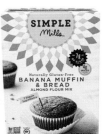 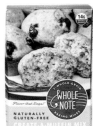 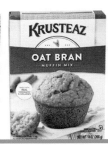 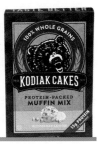

HODGSON MILL GLUTEN FREE SWEET YELLOW CORNBREAD MIX
(1 muffin)
Hodgson Mills uses **100 percent** cornmeal and is half as sweet.
CALORIES 110
SUGAR 4 g
(1 tsp)

SIMPLE MILLS BANANA MUFFIN & BREAD MIX
(1 muffin)
Almond flour subs in for white flour, and "real bananas" keep the added sugar in check.
CALORIES 90
SUGAR 7 g
(1¾ tsp)

WHOLE NOTE CREATE-A-MUFFIN MIX
(1 muffin)
Prepare as directed and you have vanilla muffins or create your own variations by adding berries.
CALORIES 120
SUGAR 11 g
(2¾ tsp)

KRUSTEAZ OAT BRAN MUFFIN MIX
(1 muffin)
These double-oat muffins are sweetened with just a touch of molasses.
CALORIES 180
SUGAR 14 g
(3½ tsp)

KODIAK CAKES BLUEBERRY LEMON MUFFIN MIX
(1 muffin)
You'll get 15 g of protein in each 100 percent whole-grain muffin.
CALORIES 120
SUGAR 11 g
(2¾ tsp)

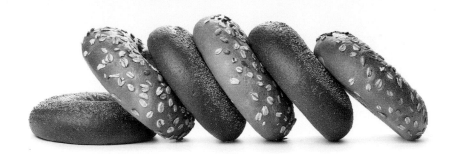

The Facts: Bagels and Your Sugar Belly

If you love a toasted bagel in the morning or you like to split one for a sandwich, know this: Your favorite bagel is most likely supersized, a hefty source of refined white flour, and a high-GI food that can cause powerful spikes in blood sugar.

FACT America is bagel-crazy. According to Statista, a statistics resource for the American food retail industry, the U.S. consumption of bagels steadily increased over the past decade and is projected to reach nearly 213 million a year by 2020.

FACT According to the National Institutes of Health, 20 years ago, a standard bagel was just three inches in diameter and had 140 calories. Today, a medium-size plain bagel can be six inches in diameter and contain 350 calories.

FACT Many brands of bagels have been processed by food manufacturers so that the whole grain is no longer intact. While these bagels have "enriched" on the label (meaning some nutrients are added back during production), they are often still lacking in fiber—an important nutrient that helps control blood sugar.

FACT Bagels are more dense than bread. A supersize bagel from a bakery or bagel shop can be equivalent to eating four to six slices of bread. So even if you order a whole wheat bagel, you can count on it raising your blood sugar.

The Fix: Build a Better Bagel

Good news: There are ways you can make your bagel healthier.

FIX **Eat just half a bagel.** Less bagel, fewer empty calories and sugar.

FIX **Choose whole-grain bagels**, versus bagels made with refined white flour and zero fiber.

FIX **Limit sweet bagels** (e.g., cinnamon-raisin and swirl bagels) to an occasional treat. Check the ingredients and choose brands without corn syrup or other added sweeteners.

FIX **Spread with filling, high-protein toppings.** Rather than reaching for the cream cheese, which comes with more than one gram (¼ teaspoon) of added sugar in every ounce, choose high-protein toppings like nut butter, smoked salmon, hummus, or a scrambled egg—they will help fill you up and prevent you from going for that other bagel half.

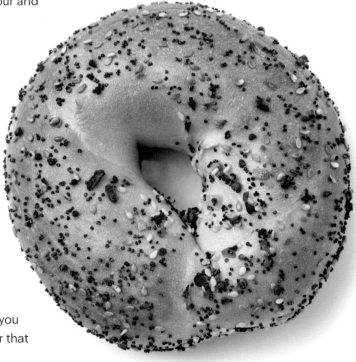

RESTAURANT BAGELS

Don't expect a petite-size bagel from a fast-food or casual restaurant—
and if it's sweet, count on heaps of added sugar.

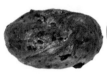 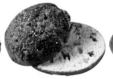  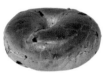 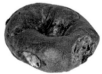

PANERA CRANBERRY WALNUT BAGEL (1 bagel)	EINSTEIN BROS APPLE CINNAMON BAGEL (1 bagel)	PANERA CINNAMON CRUNCH BAGEL (1 bagel)	BRUEGGERS BLUEBERRY BAGEL (1 bagel)	DUNKIN' CINNAMON RAISIN BAGEL (1 bagel)
CALORIES 340	**CALORIES** 450	**CALORIES** 420	**CALORIES** 310	**CALORIES** 320
SUGAR 14 g (3½ tsp)	**SUGAR** 30 g (7½ tsp)	**SUGAR** 33 g (8¼ tsp)	**SUGAR** 14 g (3½ tsp)	**SUGAR** 13 g (3¼ tsp)

More sugar than fifteen slices of white bread!

SMART SWAP
RESTAURANT BAGEL

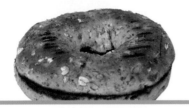 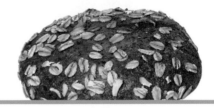

Sugar Shock   →   **Smart Swap**
CHICK-FIL-A SUNFLOWER   **PANERA SPROUTED**
MULTIGRAIN BAGEL   **GRAIN BAGEL FLAT**
(1 bagel)   (1 bagel)

As if table sugar isn't   A more reasonable size helps
enough in this bagel, Chick-fil-A   keep the added sugar in check.
adds brown sugar too.   **CALORIES** 180

CALORIES 290   **SUGAR** 4 g (1 tsp)

SUGAR 8 g (2 tsp)

SMART SWAP
STORE-BOUGHT BAGEL

Supermarket bagels may not be as super-sized as their restaurant brethren, but they're still a problem if you're keeping tabs on added sugar.

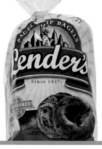

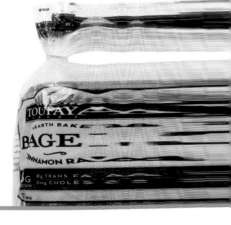

Sugar Shock
LENDER'S CINNAMON RAISIN SWIRL BAGELS
(1 bagel)
Lender's Bagels are sweetened with high-fructose corn syrup.
CALORIES 220
SUGAR 10 g (2½ tsp)

→

Smart Sw
TOUFAYAN CIN
RAISIN SMART
(1 bagel)
The thin size of t
means you can enjoy
with far less add
CALORIES
SUGAR 2 g (

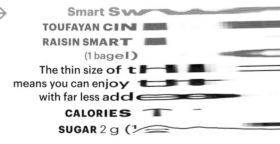

SMART SWAP
RESTAURANT BAGEL

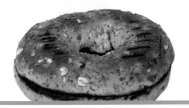 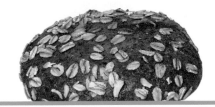

Sugar Shock	→	Smart Swap

Sugar Shock
CHICK-FIL-A SUNFLOWER
MULTIGRAIN BAGEL
(1 bagel)

As if table sugar isn't enough in this bagel, Chick-fil-A adds brown sugar too.

CALORIES 290

SUGAR 8 g (2 tsp)

Smart Swap
PANERA SPROUTED
GRAIN BAGEL FLAT
(1 bagel)

A more reasonable size helps keep the added sugar in check.

CALORIES 180

SUGAR 4 g (1 tsp)

SMART SWAP
STORE-BOUGHT BAGELS

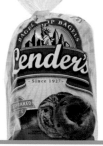

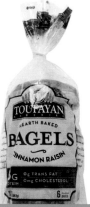

Sugar Shock
LENDER'S CINNAMON RAISIN SWIRL BAGELS
(1 bagel)
Lender's Bagels are sweetened with high-fructose corn syrup.
CALORIES 220
SUGAR 10 g (2½ tsp)

→

Smart Swap
TOUFAYAN CINNAMON RAISIN SMART BAGELS
(1 bagel)
The thin size of this bagel means you can enjoy the raisins but with far less added sugar.
CALORIES 100
SUGAR 2 g (½ tsp)

FIVE HEALTHY
PLAIN BAGELS

What makes these bagels fab? They're plain, so you can use them for breakfast or lunch. Plus, none contain more than 1¼ teaspoons of added sugar.

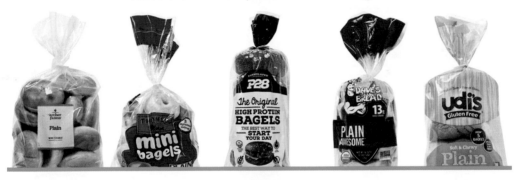

ARCHER FARMS PLAIN MINI BAGELS
(1 mini bagel)
Target's minis have the lowest amount of added sugar on the market.
CALORIES 100
SUGAR 1 g
(¼ tsp)

THOMAS' PLAIN MINI BAGELS
(1 mini bagel)
You won't fine high-fructose corn syrup in these minis.
CALORIES 125
SUGAR 3 g
(¾ tsp)

P28 HIGH PROTEIN PLAIN BAGELS
(1 bagel)
Not only are there 28 g of protein per bagel, but you'll also get 4 grams of fiber.
CALORIES 260
SUGAR 5 g
(1¼ tsp)

DAVE'S KILLER BREAD PLAIN AWESOME BAGELS
(1 bagel)
One bagel delivers 13 g of whole grains, including quinoa, spelt, rye, millet, and barley.
CALORIES 260
SUGAR 5 g
(1¼ tsp)

UDI'S GLUTEN FREE PLAIN BAGELS
(1 bagel)
These soft and chewy bagels are a good pick if you want to go gluten free.
CALORIES 290
SUGAR 5 g
(1¼ tsp)

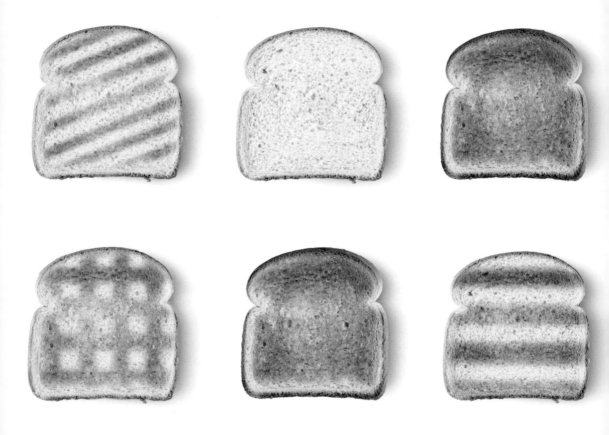

The Facts: Bread and Sugar

Ready to make a sammie? Think twice before you reach for your favorite store-bought bread, because it most likely contains added sugar. While a few grams of sweet per slice might not seem to be a big deal, it's double that number for a sandwich. We help you find the breads that don't rely on added sugar for their great taste.

FACT Sugar is not an essential ingredient in bread. However, it's added to the majority of commercial breads to retain moisture, add softness, and accommodate Americans' taste for sweet.

FACT Beware of breads that claim to be "whole-grain, whole wheat, or white-wheat" without adding a percentage on the label. Currently, the USDA has very few regulations for whole-grain labeling, according to the Whole Grains Council, a nonprofit consumer advocacy group. Whole grains provide more fiber, vitamins, minerals, and important nutrients than refined grains. That means bread manufacturers can mix in a small amount of whole wheat with refined white flour and place healthy-sounding words like "multigrain" on their packaging, which may mislead consumers.

FACT "One-hundred percent natural" bread doesn't mean it's whole wheat or whole-grain. Breads labeled "7-grain" might have seven grains but may also contain a fair amount of refined flour.

FACT If the first ingredient is "enriched wheat flour," this is primarily white bread. Some nutrients are added back in, but it is not the same as a whole-grain product.

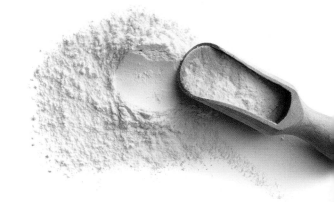

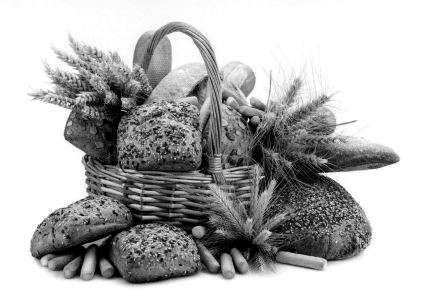

The Fix: A Better Slice

Given the hundreds of different packaged breads to choose from at the supermarket, it can be a challenge to leave with a healthy loaf. The good news is that the nutrition and ingredient labels are your best friend. These tips will help you choose the best-for-you low-sugar bread.

FIX Buy bread with a percentage of whole-grain versus plain old white bread. Whole grains provide higher amounts of fiber and protein, both of which slow the absorption of sugar in your bloodstream to keep blood sugar steady. **SOLA Golden Wheat Low Carb Sandwich Bread** has just 1 gram (¼ teaspoon) of sugar per slice.

FIX Choose bread with no more than two grams of added sugar per slice. Remember, you'll double that when you make a sandwich. If you're having trouble finding a loaf without added sugar, keep in mind that ingredients are listed by weight. The farther down sugar is listed on the ingredient list, the less the bread will contain.

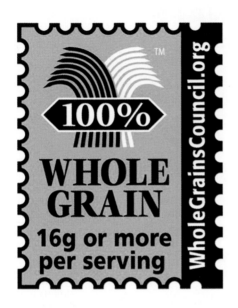

• **100% Stamp** All the grain ingredients are whole grain. Each serving contains a minimum of 16 grams of whole grains per serving.

• **50%+ Stamp** At least half the grain ingredients are whole grain, with a minimum of eight grams of whole grain per serving.

• **Basic Stamp Bread** contains at least eight grams of whole grain but may contain more refined grain than whole.

NOTE: If a product contains large amounts of whole grain (such as over 23 grams) but also contains extra bran, germ, or refined flour, it will use the 50%+ Stamp or the Basic Stamp (and not the 100% Stamp).

FIX **Select breads with at least two to three grams of fiber and three to five grams of protein per slice.**

FIX **Look for the "Whole Grain Stamp" on packaged bread from the Whole Grains Council** (you'll find it on crackers and other baked goods too). This is an easy shortcut for finding brands that offer at least half a serving of whole grains. There are three types of stamps:

FIX **Try bread made from sprouted grains.** Sprouting is a process in which grains are repeatedly soaked and rinsed for several days to enhance their digestibility. Because sprouting partially breaks down the starch in the grains, which lowers the carbs and increases fiber content, sprouted bread has less of an impact on blood sugar compared with other brands in the bread aisle.

SMART SWAPS
BREADS

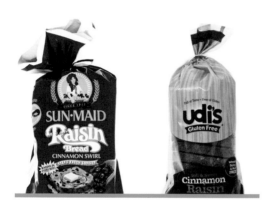

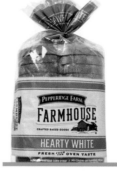

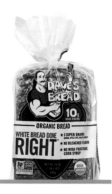

Sugar Shock →

SUN MAID RAISIN CINNAMON SWIRL BREAD

(1 slice)

Raisin juice concentrate (in addition to the raisins) is one reason why Sun Maid has the highest added sugar of any popular brand.

CALORIES 100

SUGAR 8 g (2 tsp)

Smart Swap

UDI'S GLUTEN FREE CINNAMON RAISIN BREAD

(1 slice)

Brown rice flour versus the white stuff helps keep the added sugar in check.

CALORIES 70

SUGAR 5 g (1¼ tsp)

Sugar Shock →

PEPPERIDGE FARM FARMHOUSE HEARTY WHITE BREAD

(1 slice)

While "farmhouse" may sound like better-for-you bread, that's not the case for this brand of sliced white.

CALORIES 130

SUGAR 4 g (1 tsp)

Smart Swap

DAVE'S KILLER BREAD, ORGANIC WHITE BREAD DONE RIGHT

(1 slice)

Not only does Dave's cut the added sugar, but it has the most whole grains of any packaged organic white bread.

CALORIES 110

SUGAR 2 g (½ tsp)

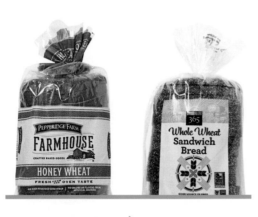
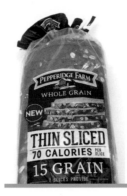
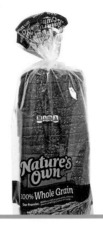

Sugar Shock →

Smart Swap

PEPPERIDGE FARM FARMHOUSE HONEY WHEAT BREAD
(1 slice)

Pepperidge Farm may be 100 percent whole wheat, but it's still sweetened with three kinds of added sugar.

CALORIES 140

SUGAR 6 g (1½ tsp)

365 EVERYDAY VALUE WHOLE WHEAT SANDWICH BREAD
(1 slice)

You can feel a lot better about making a sandwich with this Whole Foods brand.

CALORIES 100

SUGAR 2 g (½ tsp)

Sugar Shock →

Smart Swap

PEPPERIDGE FARM WHOLE GRAIN THIN SLICED 15 GRAIN BREAD
(1 slice)

Despite being "thin," added sugar is the next ingredient after whole-wheat flour and water.

CALORIES 140

SUGAR 4 g (1 tsp)

NATURE'S OWN 100% WHOLE GRAIN BREAD
(1 slice)

With half the calories, this soft sandwich bread has the Whole Grain Stamp you're looking for.

CALORIES 70

SUGAR 2 g (½ tsp)

SMART SWAPS
BREADS

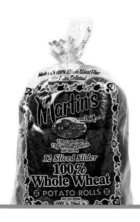
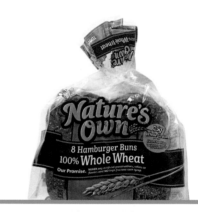

$\rightarrow$

Sugar Shock
MARTIN'S 100%
WHOLE WHEAT POTATO ROLLS
(1 roll)

These rolls may have 13 grams of whole grains, but they're also sweetened with sugar and cane sugar syrup.

CALORIES 100
SUGAR 4 g (1 tsp)

Smart Swap
NATURE'S OWN
SANDWICH 100% WHOLE WHEAT
HAMBURGER BUNS
(1 bun

Nature's Own delivers 100 percent whole grains like Martin's but with half the sweet stuff.

CALORIES 100
SUGAR 2 g (½ tsp)

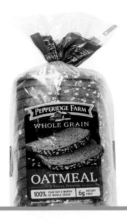

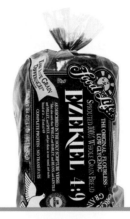

	→	
Sugar Shock		**Smart Swap**
PEPPERIDGE FARM WHOLE GRAIN OATMEAL BREAD		**EZEKIEL 4:9 SPROUTED WHOLE GRAIN BREAD**
(1 slice)		(1 slice)

Sugar Shock

PEPPERIDGE FARM WHOLE GRAIN OATMEAL BREAD

(1 slice)

While this bread is made with whole wheat flour and oats, it's still too much added sugar when there are healthier alternatives.

CALORIES 130

SUGAR 4 g (1 tsp)

Smart Swap

EZEKIEL 4:9 SPROUTED WHOLE GRAIN BREAD

(1 slice)

Fiber- and nutrient-rich sprouted grains, lentils, and soybeans make this the best bet.

CALORIES 80

SUGAR 0 g (0 tsp)

ENGLISH MUFFINS

Most English muffins have just a trace of added sugar if they're plain, like Thomas' Original, which contains less than one gram of added sweet. But when you factor in added flavors, even multigrain English muffins can be too sugary.

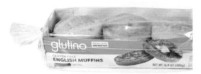

GLUTINO ORIGINAL GLUTEN FREE ENGLISH MUFFINS (1 muffin)
CALORIES 180 **SUGAR** 7 g (1¾ tsp)

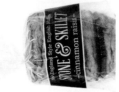

STONE & SKILLET CINNAMON RAISIN ENGLISH MUFFINS (1 muffin)
CALORIES 170 **SUGAR** 8 g (2 tsp)

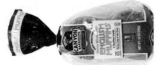

BAYS CINNAMON RAISIN ENGLISH MUFFINS (1 muffin)
CALORIES 170 **SUGAR** 10 g (2½ tsp)

More sugar than two mini Mr. Goodbars!

CANYON BAKE HOUSE HONEY WHOLE GRAIN ENGLISH MUFFINS (1 muffin)
CALORIES 200 **SUGAR** 5 g (1¼ tsp)

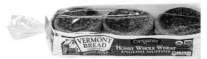

VERMONT BREAD HONEY WHEAT ORGANIC ENGLISH MUFFINS (1 muffin)
CALORIES 120 **SUGAR** 5 g (1¼ tsp)

SMART SWAP
ENGLISH MUFFINS

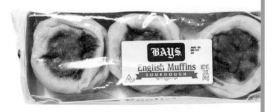

Sugar Shock
BAYS SOURDOUGH
ENGLISH MUFFINS
(1 muffin)
Fans of sourdough watch out.
These English muffins are
sweetened with cane sugar.
That's just too sweet.
CALORIES 130
SUGAR 3 g (¾ tsp)

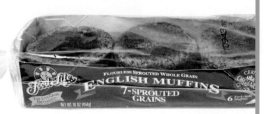

Smart Swap
FOOD FOR LIFE 7-SPROUTED
GRAINS ENGLISH MUFFINS
(1 muffin)
These muffins boast seven
sprouted grains, which help keep
your blood sugar levels in check.
CALORIES 160
SUGAR 0 g (0 tsp)

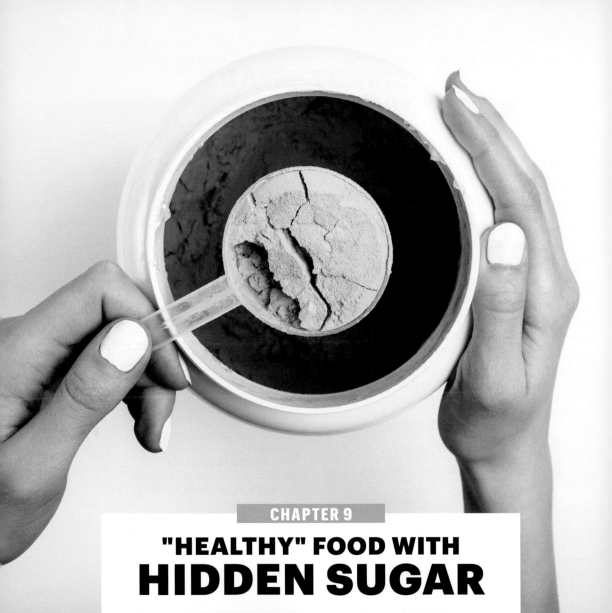

CHAPTER 9

"HEALTHY" FOOD WITH
HIDDEN SUGAR

Healthy—and Pumped Full of Sugar

These are the foods you never imagined could be sugar bombs: shockers like protein powder (shown at left), flavored yogurt, bars, veggie burgers, nut butters, and more. You choose these "healthy" items with the best of intentions—and often the nutritional benefits are legit. Unfortunately, in these products, as with all processed foods, added sugar creeps in. No worries. We've got just the strategies and smart swaps you'll need to control the sweet. The result? Next time you reach for something healthy, you'll know how to recognize the real deal.

The Facts: Not All Yogurts Are Created Equal

When you take a closer look at the sugar content of some yogurts at the supermarket, you might think you're in the dessert aisle.

FACT According to the AHA, flavored yogurt is one of the major sources of added sugar.

FACT Sales of flavored yogurt are huge. The latest retail sales in the U.S. yogurt industry was just shy of $9 billion per year according to Packaged Facts.

FACT According to the Center for Science in the Public Interest, consumers may get 25 percent or more of the daily recommended sugar limit of 24 grams (6 teaspoons) from just one serving of flavored yogurt.

FACT Plain yogurt contains lactose, a naturally occurring sugar, but the current nutrition label for flavored yogurt only lists "sugars" on the label. Until added sugars are listed separately on a new nutrition label (see page 30), it will be hard to figure the exact amount of added sweet in your flavored yogurt because the amount of lactose in plain yogurt and Greek yogurt can vary from brand to brand.

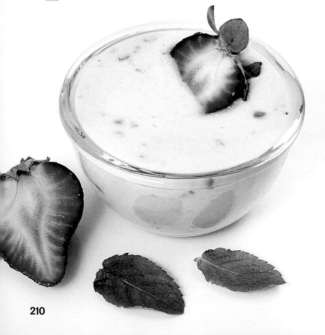

The Fix: Jazz Up Plain Yogurt

As a calcium powerhouse and a source of high-quality protein, plain yogurt deserves its health halo. That's especially true for yogurts that contain live, active bacteria cultures. These cultures, or probiotics, are considered "good bacteria" for the gut and can help maintain healthy digestive systems. But flavored yogurt is a different story. Thanks to these fixes, it's easy to enjoy the benefits of yogurt with a touch of sweet.

FIX **Sweeten plain yogurt yourself.** The difference in the amount of added sugar between plain and the presweetened stuff is huge. You're better off adding a teaspoon of honey or maple syrup to half a cup of plain yogurt.

FIX **Add fruit (versus jam) to plain yogurt.** This way you get more fiber and know that real fruit is going in as well, without the sugar added in manufacturing.

FIX **Add cinnamon to plain yogurt.** You'll add flavor without sugar.

FIX **If you can't give up flavored yogurt, limit yourself to 12 grams of sugar (or less) per serving.** That's three teaspoons of the sweet stuff.

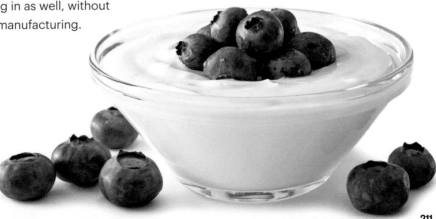

SUGAR HALL OF SHAME
FLAVORED YOGURTS

With numbers as high as these, you might
as well be eating ice cream.

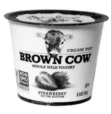

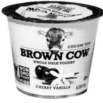

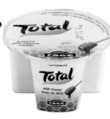

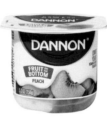

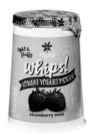

BROWN COW WHOLE MILK YOGURT, STRAWBERRY ON THE BOTTOM
(5.3 oz)

CALORIES 160
SUGAR 22 g
(5½ tsp)

BROWN COW YOGURT, CHERRY VANILLA
(5.3 oz)

CALORIES 160
SUGAR 23 g
(5¾ tsp)

FAGE TOTAL YOGURT, HONEY
(5.3 oz)

CALORIES 210
SUGAR 29 g
(7¼ tsp)

DANNON FRUIT ON THE BOTTOM, PEACH
(5.3 oz)

CALORIES 130
SUGAR 22 g
(5½ tsp)

YOPLAIT WHIPS! LOWFAT YOGURT MOUSSE, STRAWBERRY MIST
(4 oz)

CALORIES 140
SUGAR 21 g
(5¼ tsp)

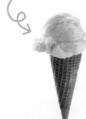

More sugar than ½ cup vanilla ice cream!

SMART SWAP
FLAVORED YOGURT

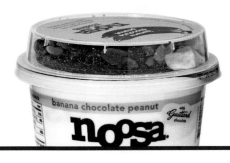
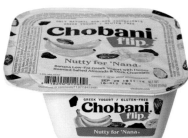

Sugar Shock	→	**Smart Swap**
NOOSA MATES, BANANA CHOCOLATE PEANUT		CHOBANI FLIP, NUTTY FOR 'NANA
(5.8 oz)		(5.3 oz)
The only real fruit you'll find in this yogurt with toppings are banana powder and sweetened banana chips.		Chobani delivers the same chocolate crunch topping but with far less added sugar.
CALORIES 280		**CALORIES** 200
SUGAR 26 g (6½ tsp)		**SUGAR** 14 g (3½ tsp)

SMART SWAPS
FLAVORED YOGURTS

Watch out! Beware of cartoon characters marketing sugar products to kids.

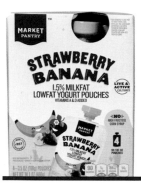
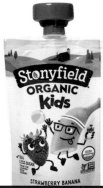
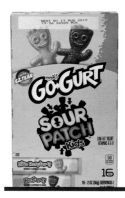
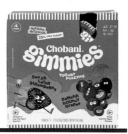

Sugar Shock →

MARKET PANTRY STRAWBERRY BANANA LOWFAT YOGURT POUCHES

(1 pouch)

This brand from Target is a tad too sweet.

CALORIES 90

SUGAR 14 g (3½ tsp)

Smart Swap

STONYFIELD ORGANIC KIDS LOW FAT STRAWBERRY BANANA YOGURT POUCHES

(1 pouch)

Stonyfield delivers the same flavor, but it's organic and less sugary.

CALORIES 90

SUGAR 9 g (2¼ tsp)

Sugar Shock →

YOPLAIT GO GURT SOUR PATCH KIDS, BLUE RASPBERRY/ REDBERRY

(1 tube)

Too many "added flavors" and way too much sugar per tube.

CALORIES 50

SUGAR 8 g (2 tsp)

Smart Swap

CHOBANI GIMMIES SUPERBERRY ROCKET YOGURT TUBES

(1 tube)

This superhero pick has no artificial flavors or preservatives.

CALORIES 40

SUGAR 4 g (1 tsp)

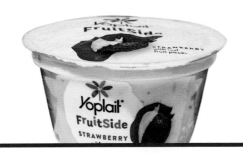
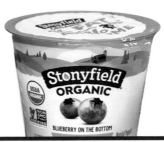

Sugar Shock

YOPLAIT FRUITSIDE,
STRAWBERRY

(5.3 oz)

While there are "real fruit pieces" on the sweet side of this yogurt, it's still strawberry preserves.

CALORIES 160

SUGAR 19 g (4¾ tsp)

Smart Swap

STONYFIELD ORGANIC
0% YOGURT,
BLUEBERRY ON THE BOTTOM

(5.3 oz)

Same berry flavor, but organic and fewer calories.

CALORIES 90

SUGAR 14 g (3½ tsp)

SMART SWAP
FLAVORED YOGURT

 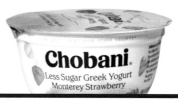

Sugar Shock		Smart Swap
NOOSA STRAWBERRY RHUBARB YOGURT		**CHOBANI LESS SUGAR MONTEREY STRAWBERRY YOGURT**
(4 oz)		(5.3 oz)
With sweetened fruit puree plus more sugar and honey, this yogurt can only be characterized as extra sweet.		Greek yogurt, which tends to be higher in protein, is more filling, plus less sugar allows the strawberry flavor to shine through.
CALORIES 140		**CALORIES** 120
SUGAR 15 g (3¾ tsp)		**SUGAR** 9 g (2¼ tsp)

FIVE LOW-SUGAR
PLAIN YOGURTS
Whether you sweeten your yogurt or not, here are
five great brands to choose from (none of which has more
than 7 grams of natural sugar).

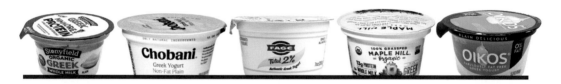

STONYFIELD ORGANIC GREEK PLAIN WHOLE MILK YOGURT	**CHOBANI PLAIN NON-FAT GREEK YOGURT**	**FAGE TOTAL 2% PLAIN GREEK YOGURT**	**MAPLE HILL CREAMERY PLAIN GREEK YOGURT**	**DANNON OIKOS GREEK NONFAT YOGURT, PLAIN**
(5.37 oz)	(5.3 oz)	(7 oz)	(5.3 oz)	(5.3 oz)
It's made with organic non-GMO, pasture-raised milk.	If you're going with fat-free yogurt, Chobani is a higher-protein pick.	While it's not organic, Fage is impressively high in protein, packing in 20 grams per single-serve container.	Maple Hill is made with grass-fed milk, which is higher in omega-3s, a nutrient linked to improved heart health.	The 15 grams of protein per serving will help keep you full for hours.
CALORIES 130	**CALORIES** 80	**CALORIES** 140	**CALORIES** 140	**CALORIES** 80
SUGAR 4 g	**SUGAR** 4 g	**SUGAR** 6 g	**SUGAR** 7 g	**SUGAR** 6 g
(1 tsp)	(1 tsp)	(1½ tsp)	(1¾ tsp)	(1½ tsp)

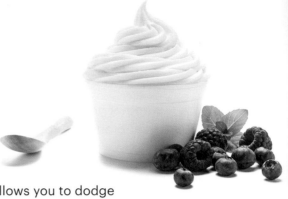

The Facts: Fro-Yo and Sugar

Choosing frozen yogurt over ice cream allows you to dodge some fat and calories. But when it comes to added sugar, don't be fooled. Your favorite fro-yo is not automatically healthier.

FACT Manufacturers add more sugar to frozen yogurt than to ice cream. The average amount of added sugar in a half-cup of fro-yo is about 17 grams (4¼ teaspoons), versus 13 grams (3¼ teaspoons) for the same amount of ice cream.

FACT Toppings are notoriously high in sugar. Even healthier-sounding toppings like fruit sauce or granola can quickly pack on extra calories and fat. According to a study in the Journal of Consumer Psychology, people who add what they perceive as "healthy" toppings to foods not only underestimate their caloric content but also eat more of the food.

FACT Frozen yogurt is not the same as fresh yogurt and does not offer the same healthful benefits. Fresh yogurt contains probiotics, a type of bacteria that helps prevent digestive problems and also boosts your immune system (see page 211). However, probiotics do not survive in cold temperatures, so they're lost in the freezing process.

FACT According to a survey conducted by Menchie's, North America's largest self-serve frozen yogurt franchise, 95 percent of Americans believe fro-yo is better for them than ice cream.

The Fix: A Healthier Frozen Yogurt

Our fixes will transform your next frozen yogurt from a sugar bomb to a healthy treat.

FIX Choose low-fat frozen yogurt over fat-free at the yogurt shop. Manufacturers usually add more sugar to fat-free fro-yo to compensate for its lack of flavor and texture. Frozen yogurt containing some fat can also slow the body's digestion of sugar, meaning you'll feel more satisfied and won't experience a blood sugar spike.

FIX Ask for the smallest cup at the fro-yo shop (they may not be on display) and cap your portion at four or five ounces max. Have your portion weighed at the counter before you add any toppings.

FIX Minimize the toppers. When sugary toppers are served salad-bar style at the fro-yo bar, it's incredibly easy to go overboard. In fact, the fro-yo sellers count on you to pile on the toppings, because they sell their products by weight. So stick to no more than two of those little black scoops. (For more about fro-yo toppings, see next page.) Better yet, go for naked fro-yo.

FIX Limit your portion of packaged frozen yogurt to half a cup. That's about the size of a baseball or your fist.

FIX Look for the "Live and Active Cultures" seal on packaged frozen yogurt and at the yogurt shop. To compensate for the loss of active cultures during freezing, some manufacturers add extra probiotics after production. This seal, created by the National Yogurt Association, confirms that a product has 100 million cultures per gram, which, among other health benefits, can help lactose-intolerant people digest milk-based products.

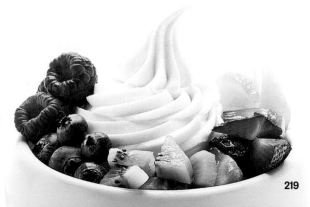

Be a Smart Topper

Going out for fro-yo is the clean eater's alternative to hitting the ice-cream parlor. A half-cup of plain frozen yogurt is pretty innocent as far as splurges go—until you start piling on the extras. While a sprinkle of this or that might not seem like a big deal, top your fro-yo with two tablespoons of caramel syrup, 17 mini gummy bears, and two tablespoons of Fruity Pebbles cereal and the amount of added sugar will increase by a whopping 43 grams (10¾ teaspoons). Here's what you can do to keep your frozen treat from turning into an ice-cream sundae.

• **BEWARE OF GRANOLA.** Oats, nuts, and dried fruit have health benefits, but when you bake them all together with loads of fat and sugar for granola, you get a super-calorie-dense topper (for more about granola, see page 158). If you want to add some granola-like flavor to your fro-yo, try a scoop of chopped nuts and half a scoop of dried fruit instead.

• **REPLACE THE FRUIT SAUCE WITH FRESH FRUIT.** That sweet, gooey liquid bathing your strawberries, pineapple, or kiwifruit is pure sugar—and those vivid colors likely come from artificial food dye. In fact, 2 tablespoons of strawberry sauce has 21 grams (5¼ teaspoons) of sugar, whereas an entire cup of chopped fresh strawberries has half the calories and seven grams (1¾ teaspoons) of naturally occurring sugar.

• **ADD FRESH FRUIT FIRST.** Choose bigger fruits like whole strawberries, raspberries, and blueberries—they'll help your cup look fuller—then head to the machine and add your fro-yo. If you still want to top it off, go with less sugary choices like unsweetened coconut flakes.

• **CHOOSE CHOPPED DARK CHOCOLATE INSTEAD OF CHOCOLATE SAUCE OR CRUSHED OREOS.** Dark chocolate contains far less sugar and is a good source of antioxidants. Plus, you won't need much (half a scoop) to get your chocolate fix.

FIVE LESS-SUGARY PICKS

AT THE FROZEN YOGURT SHOP

Best enjoyed no more than once a week, these fro-yos have the lowest added sugar on the menu.

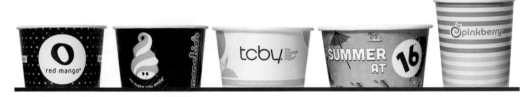

RED MANGO CREAMY PEANUT BUTTER FROZEN YOGURT	MENCHIE'S ORIGINAL TART FROZEN YOGURT	TCBY GREEK HONEY VANILLA FROZEN YOGURT	16 HANDLES YO SOY VANILLA FROZEN YOGURT	PINKBERRY ORANGE PEACH MANGO FROZEN YOGURT
(½ cup)	(½ cup)	(½ cup)	(⅔ cup)	(½ cup)
Made with natural peanut butter and a quarter less sweet than the brand's vanilla yogurt.	This tangy pick starts with fat-free milk.	Each serving delivers eight grams of protein.	This soy milk–based treat is a great choice for vegans.	This low-fat fro-yo bursts with fruit flavor.
CALORIES 130	**CALORIES** 90	**CALORIES** 100	**CALORIES** 147	**CALORIES** 90
SUGAR 18 g	**SUGAR** 15 g	**SUGAR** 13 g	**SUGAR** 12 g	**SUGAR** 18 g
(4½ tsp)	(3¾ tsp)	(3¼ tsp)	(3 tsp)	(4½ tsp)

SMART SWAPS
FROZEN YOGURTS

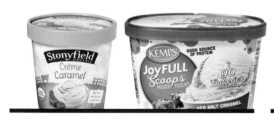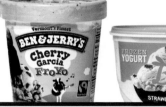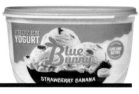

Sugar Shock →	**Smart Swap**
STONYFIELD ORGANIC CRÈME CARAMEL FROZEN LOW FAT YOGURT	**KEMP'S JOYFULL SCOOPS FROZEN YOGURT, SEA SALT CARAMEL**
(½ cup)	(⅔ cup)
Stonyfield may be organic, but its line of frozen yogurts are among the sweetest of all major brands.	If caramel is your thing, Kemp's delivers the same fabulous taste with only a fraction of the sugar.
CALORIES 140	**CALORIES** 110
SUGAR 26 g (6½ tsp)	**SUGAR** 10 g (2½ tsp)

Sugar Shock →	**Smart Swap**
BEN & JERRY'S CHERRY GARCIA FROYO	**BLUE BUNNY STRAWBERRY BANANA FROZEN YOGURT**
(⅔ cup)	(½ cup)
Too bad this fave from Ben & Jerry's comes with a hefty amount of added sugar.	If you're looking for a low-fat frozen yogurt that's less sweet, this one's for you.
CALORIES 230	**CALORIES** 100
SUGAR 29 g (7¼ tsp)	**SUGAR** 16 g (4 tsp)

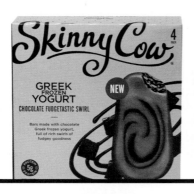

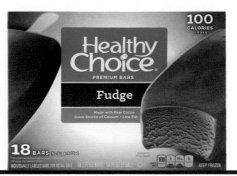

Sugar Shock

SKINNY COW CHOCOLATE
FUDGETASTIC SWIRL FROZEN
GREEK YOGURT BARS

(1 bar)

These may have 5 grams of protein but
also have three kinds of added sugar.

CALORIES 150

SUGAR 13 g (3¼ tsp)

→

Smart Swap

HEALTHY CHOICE FROZEN
FUDGE BARS

(1 bar)

For less sweet, these treats also
pack a protein punch.

CALORIES 100

SUGAR 5 g (1¼ tsp)

SUGAR HALL OF SHAME

NUTRITION BARS

There are dozens and dozens of nutrition bars promising everything from "meal replacement" to "sustained energy" to "protein." But what's missing on the label? That's simple: Most nutrition bars have as much added sugar as candy.

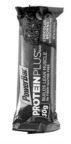

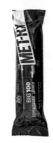

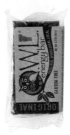

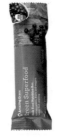

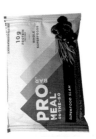

POWER BAR PROTEIN PLUS CHOCOLATE BROWNIE
(1 bar)

CALORIES 330
SUGAR 27 g
(6¾ tsp)

MET-RX BIG 100 SUPER COOKIE CRUNCH MEAL REPLACEMENT BAR
(100 g)

CALORIES 410
SUGAR 27 g
(6¾ tsp)

O.W.L. ORIGINAL ENERGY BAR
(2.7 oz)

CALORIES 335
SUGAR 28 g
(7 tsp)

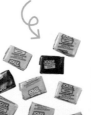

More sugar than nine Jolly Rancher Fruit Chews.

AMAZING GRASS GREEN SUPERFOOD WHOLE FOOD NUTRITION BAR, ORIGINAL
(2.1 oz)

CALORIES 220
SUGAR 24 g
(6 tsp)

PRO BAR SUPERFOOD SLAM
(85 g)

CALORIES 350
SUGAR 24 g
(6 tsp)

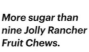

How to Pick a Healthy Nutrition Bar

Use these guidelines if don't want your nutrition bar to be a candy bar in disguise.

• **NO MORE THAN 13 GRAMS (3¼ TEASPOONS) OF SUGAR.** This should be mostly from ingredients with natural sugar, like dried fruit, not added sugars like honey or syrups.

• **A RANGE OF 150 TO 250 CALORIES.** That's the recommendation from the Academy of Nutrition and Dietetics.

• **AT LEAST SEVEN GRAMS OF PROTEIN.** That's about the same amount as in a hard-cooked egg. Nuts and nut butter are great sources of protein.

• **A MINIMUM OF THREE GRAMS OF FIBER.** Bars with fiber-rich whole grains are more filling and will help keep sugar levels in check.

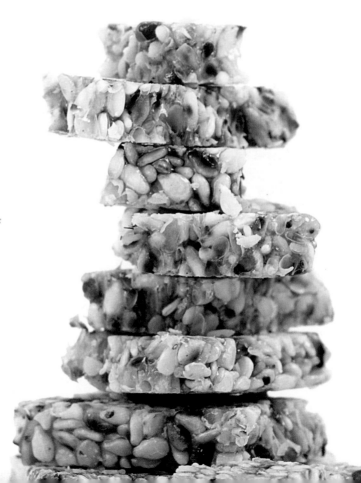

SMART SWAPS
NUTRITION BARS

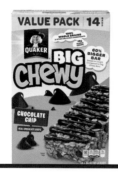
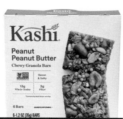
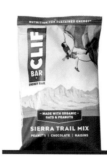
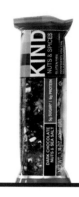

Sugar Shock →

QUAKER BIG CHEWY GRANOLA BAR, CHOCOLATE CHIP

(42 g)

Six kinds of added sugar is not what you want in your granola bar.

CALORIES 180

SUGAR 13 g (3¼ tsp)

Smart Swap

KASHI CHEWY GRANOLA BARS, PEANUT PEANUT BUTTER

(1 bar)

Each filling bar contains 13 whole grains and three grams of fiber.

CALORIES 140

SUGAR 6 g (1½ tsp)

Sugar Shock →

CLIF SIERRA TRAIL MIX ENERGY BAR

(68 g)

Brown rice syrup, cane syrup, and cane sugar are not what you need for energy, even when it's organic.

CALORIES 250

SUGAR 22 g (5½ tsp)

Smart Swap

KIND BAR DARK CHOCOLATE, NUTS & SEA SALT

(1.4 oz)

This mix of protein-rich nuts and unsweetened dried fruits ensures you'll power through your workout without a sugar crash in the middle.

CALORIES 180

SUGAR 5 g (1¼ tsp)

FIVE LOW-SUGAR
NUTRITION BARS

Check out these less sugary picks—each with less than three teaspoons of sweet.

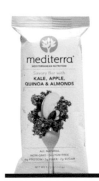 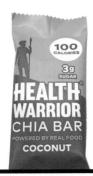 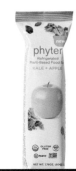 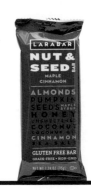 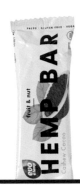

MEDITERRA SAVORY BAR WITH KALE, POMEGRANATE, QUINOA & ALMONDS	**HEALTH WARRIOR COCONUT CHIA BAR**	**PHYTER KALE + APPLE PLANT-BASED FOOD BAR**	**LARABAR MAPLE CINNAMON NUT & SEED BAR**	**EVO HEMP CASHEW CACAO BAR**
(35 g)	(25 g)	(50 g)	(1.24 oz)	(1.7 oz)
This Mediterranean-inspired bar is a savory treat.	These plant-powered bars contain a blend of protein-rich chia seeds, oats, quinoa, and peas.	This gluten-free bar offers a short list of ingredients. The flavor will remind you of apple pie.	Only eight ingredients make up this filling bar, including almonds, chia seeds, sunflower seeds, coconut oil, cinnamon, and sea salt.	The first three ingredients in this bar—dates, cashews, and apricots—are all whole foods, plus it is vegan!
CALORIES 130	**CALORIES** 100	**CALORIES** 200	**CALORIES** 210	**CALORIES** 185
SUGAR 3 g	**SUGAR** 3 g	**SUGAR** 7 g	**SUGAR** 7 g	**SUGAR** 10 g
(¾ tsp)	(¾ tsp)	(1¾ tsp)	(1¾ tsp)	(2"½ tsp)

SMART SWAP

APPLESAUCE

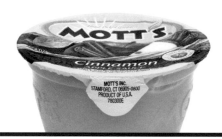 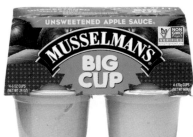

Sugar Shock		Smart Swap
MOTT'S CINNAMON APPLESAUCE		**MUSSELMAN'S UNSWEETENED APPLE SAUCE CUPS**
(4 oz cup)		(4 oz cup)

While you won't see "sweetened" on this label, don't be fooled. Like the vast majority of regular applesauces from major brands, this cup contains a hefty dose of HFCS (sucrose is another common sweetener).

CALORIES 100
SUGAR 24 g (6 tsp)

Musselman's is non-GMO verified, and the sugar is just naturally occurring fructose. Plus, the individual snack-size cup counts as one of your daily fruit servings, as recommended by the USDA's Dietary Guidelines.

CALORIES 50
SUGAR 11 g (2¾ tsp)

SMART SWAPS
NUT BUTTERS

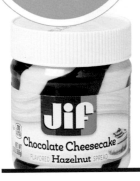

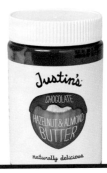

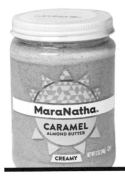

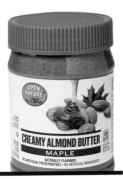

Sugar Shock →
JIF CHOCOLATE CHEESECAKE HAZELNUT SPREAD

(2 Tbsp)

You know you're in trouble when sugar is the first ingredient.

CALORIES 220

SUGAR 21 g (5¼ tsp)

Smart Swap
JUSTIN'S CHOCOLATE HAZELNUT & ALMOND SPREAD

(2 Tbsp)

Unlike Jif, this less-sugary sweet spread doesn't have any artificial ingredients.

CALORIES 200

SUGAR 8 g (2 tsp)

Sugar Shock →
MARANATHA CARAMEL ALMOND SPREAD

(2 Tbsp)

The latest addition to this "decadent line of indulgent spreads" certainly has an excess of added sugar.

CALORIES 190

SUGAR 11 g (2¾ tsp)

Smart Swap
OPEN NATURE MAPLE CREAMY ALMOND BUTTER

(2 Tbsp)

More nuts and less sugar make this supermarket brand a better bet.

CALORIES 180

SUGAR 5 g (1¼ tsp)

SMART SWAPS
NUT BUTTERS

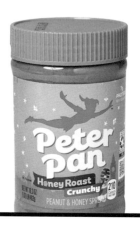
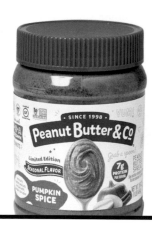

Sugar Shock
**PETER PAN CRUNCHY
PEANUT & HONEY SPREAD**

(2 Tbsp)

The honey may be organic,
but it's still added sugar.

CALORIES 210

SUGAR 7 grams (1"¾ tsp)

→

Smart Swap
**PEANUT BUTTER & CO PUMPKIN
SPICE PEANUT BUTTER SPREAD**

(2 Tbsp)

Real pumpkin, cinnamon,
nutmeg, ginger, and allspice help
keep the added sugar in check.

CALORIES 180

SUGAR 4 grams (1 tsp)

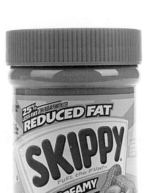

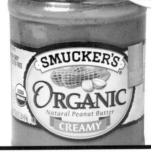

Numerous studies show that people who regularly include nuts or peanut butter in their diets are less likely to develop heart disease or type 2 diabetes than those who rarely eat nuts.

Sugar Shock → **Smart Swap**

SKIPPY REDUCED FAT CREAMY PEANUT BUTTER SPREAD

(2 Tbsp)

When peanut butter is labeled "reduced fat," it often contains the same amount of (if not more) calories, plus corn syrup.

CALORIES 190

SUGAR 4 grams (1 tsp)

SMUCKER'S ORGANIC CREAMY PEANUT BUTTER

(2 Tbsp)

The only ingredients in this jar are roasted peanuts and salt.

CALORIES 180

SUGAR 1 gram (¼ tsp)

SMART SWAPS
VEGGIE BURGERS

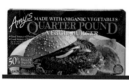
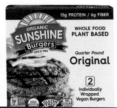
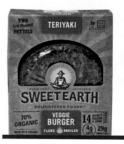
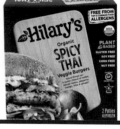

Sugar Shock →

AMY'S QUARTER POUND VEGGIE BURGER

(1 patty)

To get "the perfect hint of barbecue flavor," Amy's includes sugar and molasses in its list of ingredients.

CALORIES 210

SUGAR 6 g (1½ tsp)

Smart Swap

ORGANIC SUNSHINE BURGERS, QUARTER POUND ORIGINAL

(1 patty)

The only other ingredients you'll find in these brown rice burgers are sunflower seeds, carrots, chives, and sea salt.

CALORIES 360

SUGAR 3 g (¾ tsp)

Sugar Shock →

SWEET EARTH TERIYAKI VEGGIE BURGER

(1 patty)

If you enjoy an Asian-style burger, it's best to skip the sugary teriyaki sauce.

CALORIES 220

SUGAR 5 g (1"¼ tsp)

Smart Swap

HILARY'S ORGANIC SPICY THAI VEGGIE BURGERS

(1 patty)

Carrot, mango, ginger, and mint lend just the right amount of subtle sweetness to these spicy burgers.

CALORIES 160

SUGAR 1 g (¼ tsp)

FIVE LOW-SUGAR
VEGGIE BURGERS

These tasty burgers go from sugar-free to
no more than ¾ teaspoon of sweet.

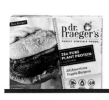
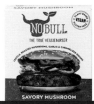
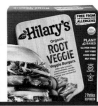
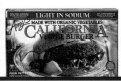

DR. PRAEGER'S ALL AMERICAN VEGGIE BURGERS

(1 patty)

With 28 grams of plant protein and 4 grams of fiber, this burger has the goods to keep you satisfied.

CALORIES 240

SUGAR 0 g

(0 tsp)

NO BULL SAVORY MUSHROOM BURGER

(1 patty)

With 10 grams of protein from lentils, quinoa, and chia seeds, this burger is practically a meal in itself.

CALORIES 170

SUGAR 1 g (¼ tsp)

HILARY'S ROOT VEGGIE BURGER

(1 patty)

Hilary's products are free of the most common food allergens in the U.S., including peanuts, milk, eggs, soy, and wheat.

CALORIES 150

SUGAR 1 g

(¼ tsp)

AMY'S CALIFORNIA VEGGIE BURGER LIGHT IN SODIUM

(1 patty)

Not only is it 50 percent lower in sodium than Amy's regular veggie burger, but it also has fewer additives.

CALORIES 150

SUGAR 1 g

(¼ tsp)

ORGANIC SUNSHINE BURGERS, BLACK BEAN SOUTH WEST

(1 patty)

Black beans supply a hefty eight grams of fiber in these vegan burgers.

CALORIES 260

SUGAR 3 g

(¾ tsp)

Sugar + Protein Powder

Before you scoop out that pro powder for your next smoothie or shake, know that you might be adding teaspoons of sugar too. Truth be told, the taste of protein powder can be bland or unpleasant. So companies add sugar to their products so they taste better (i.e. sweet). Fortunately, it's easy to make a protein-powder smoothie or shake delicious without creating a sugar bomb. Here's how:

- **AVOID SWEETENED POWDERS,** which promote weight gain. They will have more calories and sugar.
- **INCLUDE A BANANA** in your unsweetened drink. You'll be adding only natural sugar, plus potassium and vitamins.

- **ADD YOUR OWN SWEETENER** to unsweetened powder. While honey, agave nectar, and pure maple syrup are added sugars, they are less processed than the ingredients in the presweetened stuff. Plus, you'll have full control over how much sugar is in your drink.

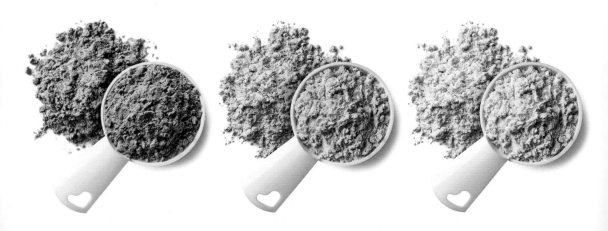

SMART SWAP
PROTEIN POWDER

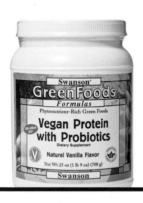 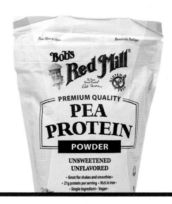

Sugar Shock

**SWANSON GREENFOODS
VEGAN PROTEIN POWDER
WITH PROBIOTICS**

(3 scoops)

Swanson combines two strains of bacteria with hemp, rice, and pea protein to create its scoopable nutrition. In theory, this all sounds like a good thing—but unfortunately, there's also a heavy dose of brown rice syrup.

CALORIES 190

SUGAR 20 g (5 tsp)

→

Smart Swap

**BOB'S RED MILL
PEA PROTEIN POWDER**

(¼ cup)

Unlike many other pea protein powders, this one has no chemical solvents—just 100 percent yellow peas and a hefty 21 grams of protein per serving.

CALORIES 100

SUGAR 0 g (0 tsp)

Sweet 'n' Chewy Vitamins

According to the latest figures from Statista, the value of gummy vitamins in the U.S. market is projected to increase from $2.5 billion to over $4 billion by 2025. And no wonder: Chewable and sweet as chewing gum, these candy-colored vitamins appeal to kids and grown-ups alike, and especially adults who deal with "pill fatigue." While gummy vitamins may be an easy way to get missing nutrients in your diet, especially if you or your kids are not eating enough fruits and veggies, it's important to keep these facts in mind:

• **THEY ARE WEAKER THAN NORMAL MULTIVITAMINS.** Due to how gummies are manufactured, gummies actually contain less vitamin content than regular multivitamins. That means they're less effective while adding sugar to your diet.

• **GUMMY VITAMINS RAISE THE RISK FOR TOOTH DECAY.** While a gram or two of sugar may not seem like a big deal, sugar in gummy form is more likely to stick to teeth, increasing the odds of bacteria growth and plaque.

• **EATING TOO MANY GUMMIES IS EASY.** Their appealing, sweet taste poses the possibility of overdoing it. Some companies are careful not to include certain nutrients that could be dangerous if taken in excess. Others, not so much.

• **VITAMIN SUPPLEMENTS ARE NOT EVALUATED FOR SAFETY AND EFFICACY BY THE USDA.** Look on the label to see if the product was tested by independent labs such as US Pharmacopeia, Consumer Lab, and NSF International. Certification ensures the labeled dosage of the correct ingredient and that there are no toxins or contaminating organisms.

According to a study from AARP, Americans over 45 say they take an average of four prescription medications a day.

SMART SWAPS
GUMMIE VITAMINS

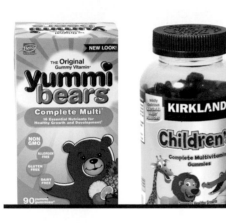

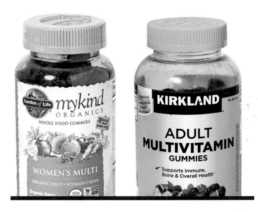

Sugar Shock → **Smart Swap**

YUMMI BEARS ORGANICS COMPLETE MULTI-VITAMIN GUMMIES

(3 bears)

Organic and non-GMO doesn't change that these gummies are supersweet.

CALORIES 25

SUGAR 5 g (1¼ tsp)

KIRKLAND SIGNATURE CHILDREN'S COMPLETE MULTIVITAMIN GUMMIES

(2 gummies)

Costco's brand is not only less sweet but also endorsed by Consumer Lab.

CALORIES 15

SUGAR 2 g (½ tsp)

Sugar Shock → **Smart Swap**

GARDEN OF LIFE MYKIND ORGANICS WOMEN'S MULTI GUMMIES

(4 gummies)

There are more calories and sugar in these adult gummies than in other leading brands.

CALORIES 35

SUGAR 5 g (1¼ tsp)

KIRKLAND SIGNATURE ADULT MULTIVITAMIN GUMMIES

(2 gummies)

Costco wins again as the most widely available lower-in-sugar gummy vitamin for adults.

CALORIES 15

SUGAR 2 g (½ tsp)

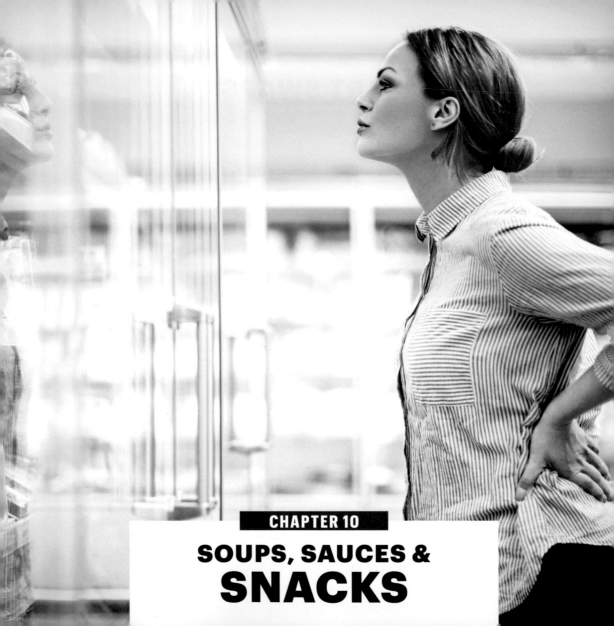

CHAPTER 10

SOUPS, SAUCES &
SNACKS

The Savory Side of Sweet

When you top spaghetti with pasta sauce, reach for a bottle of ketchup, or drizzle your salad with bottled dressing, you're probably not thinking about how much sugar you're adding to your food. After all, these are savory foods, not obvious sugar bombs like soft drinks and desserts. Unfortunately, sugar is often part of the package in the most unexpected products, especially if they're lower in fat or sodium. To help, we've trolled the supermarket aisles to reveal the most surprising items in boxes, bottles, and cans with hidden sugar. Best of all, our swaps are not only healthier, but tastier too.

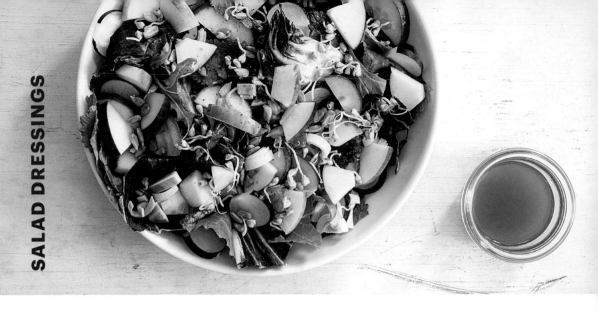

The Facts: Dressed in Sugar

If you toss your greens with the wrong type of dressing, added sugar will sneak into the salad bowl.

FACT Low-fat or fat-free salad dressings often have more sugar (and salt) than regular dressing to make up for some of the flavor that is lost when fat is removed.

FACT The standard serving size for bottled dressing is two tablespoons, but many people use much more than that, according to the Department of Nutrition at Harvard-affiliated Brigham and Women's Hospital.

FACT According to Statista, a statistics resource for the U.S. food retail industry, America's most popular dressing is ranch, which is not marketed as sweet. However, top-selling Hidden Valley Fat-Free Ranch has ¾ teaspoon sugar, or three grams per two tablespoons.

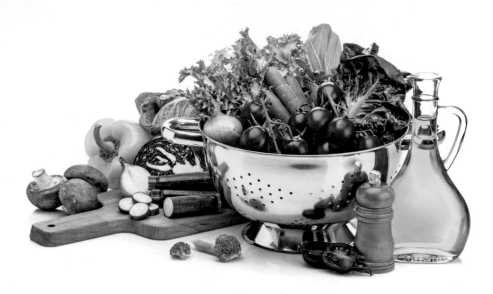

The Fix: Dress Smart

Shop and build a better, less sugary salad with these dressing fixes.

FIX Choose a dressing with no more than 120 calories, 200 grams of sodium, and 2 grams of sugar per serving. Preferred dressings should have a minimal number of ingredients and no artificial flavors or colors.

FIX If your favorite dressing exceeds these guidelines, use only half a serving (1 tablespoon). If you want more dressing, mix it with a tablespoon of balsamic, red, or white wine vinegar for vinaigrettes or water for creamy dressings.

FIX Measure dressings with measuring spoons. Eventually, you'll be able to eyeball the correct amount to keep portion control in check.

FIX Serve salad with dressing on the side and dip each bite. That will give you a blast of intense flavor with every forkful and help minimize the amount of dressing at the same time.

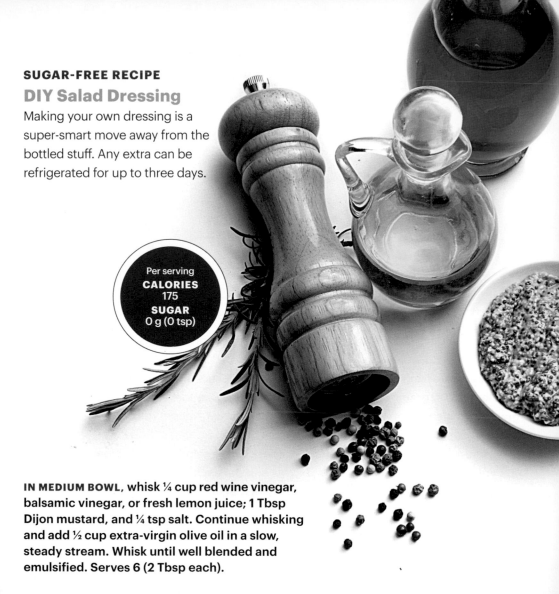

DIY Salad Dressing

Making your own dressing is a super-smart move away from the bottled stuff. Any extra can be refrigerated for up to three days.

Per serving
CALORIES
175
SUGAR
0 g (0 tsp)

IN MEDIUM BOWL, whisk ¼ cup red wine vinegar, balsamic vinegar, or fresh lemon juice; 1 Tbsp Dijon mustard, and ¼ tsp salt. Continue whisking and add ½ cup extra-virgin olive oil in a slow, steady stream. Whisk until well blended and emulsified. Serves 6 (2 Tbsp each).

SMART SWAPS
SALAD DRESSINGS

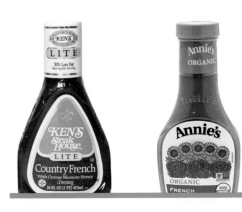
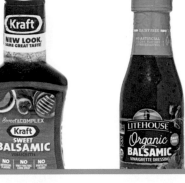

Sugar Shock →	Smart Swap	Sugar Shock →	Smart Swap
KEN'S STEAKHOUSE LITE COUNTRY FRENCH DRESSING	**ANNIE'S ORGANIC FRENCH DRESSING**	**KRAFT SWEET BALSAMIC DRESSING**	**LITEHOUSE ORGANIC BALSAMIC VINAIGRETTE DRESSING**
(2 Tbsp)	(2 Tbsp)	(2 Tbsp)	(2 Tbsp)
While Ken's light version has fewer calories, adding honey to an already sweet dressing is the wrong move.	Annie's is less sweet but still retains the flavor of the French classic.	Kraft sweetens the vinegar with grape juice to turn what is normally a subtle-tasting dressing into something too sweet.	All you'll find is organic balsamic vinegar in this dressing that has only a fraction of the sugar.
CALORIES 100	**CALORIES** 110	**CALORIES** 90	**CALORIES** 70
SUGAR 10 g (2½ tsp)	**SUGAR** 3 g (¾ tsp)	**SUGAR** 10 g (2½ tsp)	**SUGAR** 1 g (¼ tsp)

SMART SWAPS
SALAD DRESSINGS

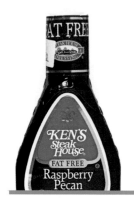 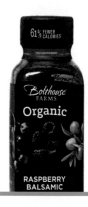 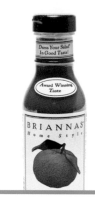 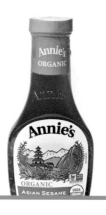

Sugar Shock →	Smart Swap	Sugar Shock →	Smart Swap
KEN'S FAT-FREE RASPBERRY PECAN DRESSING	**BOLTHOUSE FARMS ORGANIC RASPBERRY BALSAMIC VINAIGRETTE DRESSING**	**BRIANNA'S HOMESTYLE SAUCY GINGER MANDARIN DRESSING**	**ANNIE'S ORGANIC ASIAN SESAME DRESSING**
(2 Tbsp)	(2 Tbsp)	(2 Tbsp)	(2 Tbsp)
This dressing packs in artificial dyes and lists sugar as the second most abundant ingredient.	Same berry flavor but far less added sugar.	Concentrated mandarin juice and honey both jack up the sweet in this Asian dressing.	Amy's less sugary dressing features crunchy toasted sesame seeds.
CALORIES 45	**CALORIES** 35	**CALORIES** 150	**CALORIES** 130
SUGAR 10 g (2½ tsp)	**SUGAR** 3 g (¾ tsp)	**SUGAR** 8 g (2 tsp)	**SUGAR** 3 g (¾ tsp)

FIVE SUGAR-FREE
SALAD DRESSINGS
Take your pick of these healthy dressings
to toss with your next salad.

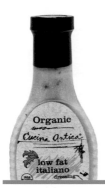
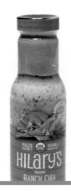
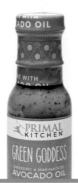
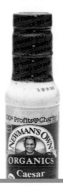
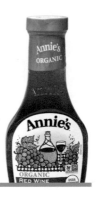

CUCINA ANTICA ORGANIC LOW-FAT ITALIANO DRESSING	**HILARY'S EAT WELL RANCH CHIA DRESSING & DIP**	**PRIMAL KITCHEN GREEN GODDESS DRESSING & MARINADE**	**NEWMAN'S OWN ORGANIC CAESAR DRESSING**	**ANNIE'S ORGANIC RED WINE & OLIVE OIL VINAIGRETTE**
(2 Tbsp)	(2 Tbsp)	(2 Tbsp)	(2 Tbsp)	(2 Tbsp)
Cucina Antica is both low-fat and sugar-free (unlike most light bottled dressings).	Hilary's concocts its creamy ranch dressing with unsweetened coconut milk.	This creamy dressing is made with avocado oil and organic herbs and spices.	Hail this Caesar dressing with no added sweet stuff.	Extra-virgin olive oil adds authentic flavor to this classic dressing.
CALORIES 30	**CALORIES** 45	**CALORIES** 120	**CALORIES** 170	**CALORIES** 140
SUGAR 0 g	**SUGAR** 0 g	**SUGAR** 0 g	**SUGAR** 0 g	**SUGAR** 0 g
(0 tsp)	(0 tsp)	(0 tsp)	(0 tsp)	(0 tsp)

PASTA SAUCES

Use these brands of bottled sauce and you might as well toss your pasta with sugar.

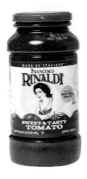

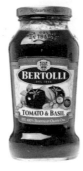

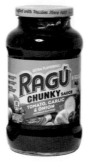

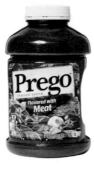

FRANCESCO RINALDI SWEET & TASTY TOMATO PASTA SAUCE
(½ cup)
CALORIES 70
SUGAR 11 g
(2¾ tsp)

BERTOLLI TOMATO & BASIL SAUCE
(½ cup)
CALORIES 80
SUGAR 11 g
(2¾ tsp)

RAGÚ CHUNKY TOMATO, GARLIC, & ONION SAUCE
(½ cup)
CALORIES 80
SUGAR 12 g
(3 tsp)

PREGO ITALIAN SAUCE WITH MEAT
(½ cup)
CALORIES 90
SUGAR 10 g
(2½ tsp)

EMERIL'S HOMESTYLE MARINARA
(½ cup)
CALORIES 90
SUGAR 9 g
(2¼ tsp)

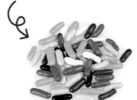

Almost as much sugar as nine Good & Plenty licorice candies.

SMART SWAP
PASTA SAUCE

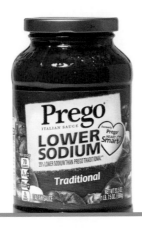 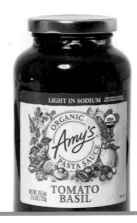

Sugar Shock	→	Smart Swap
PREGO ITALIAN SAUCE LOWER SODIUM TRADITIONAL		**AMY'S ORGANIC LIGHT IN SODIUM TOMATO BASIL**
(½ cup)		(½ cup)
To compensate for less salt, Prego adds way too much sugar.		There's no added sugar in Amy's sauce, just less sodium.
CALORIES 70		**CALORIES** 90
SUGAR 9 g (2¼ tsp)		**SUGAR** 2 g (½ tsp)

SMART SWAP
VODKA SAUCE

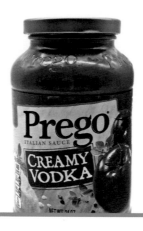
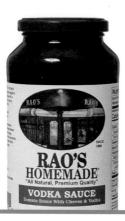

Sugar Shock
PREGO CREAMY VODKA ITALIAN SAUCE
(½ cup)

Give Prego a pass if you don't want cream and added sugar in your vodka sauce.

CALORIES 140
SUGAR 10 g (2½ tsp)

Smart Swap
RAO'S VODKA SAUCE
(½ cup)

Parmesan and pecorino cheeses sub in for cream in Rao's sauce that has no added sugar.

CALORIES 90
SUGAR 5 g (1¼ tsp)

FIVE NO-ADDED SUGAR

PASTA SAUCES

Pasta sauce without the added sweet stuff has no more than six grams of natural sugar. Here's your pick of the best.

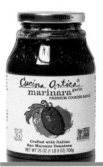 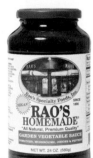 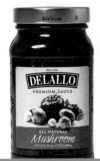 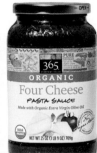 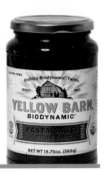

CUCINA ANTICA GARLIC MARINARA

(½ cup)

You can't go wrong with this simple marinara made with Italian San Marzano tomatoes and extra-virgin olive oil.

CALORIES 45
SUGAR 6 g
(1½ tsp)

RAO'S HOMEMADE GARDEN VEGETABLE SAUCE

(½ cup)

Tomatoes, mushrooms, bell peppers, onion, and garlic slowly simmer with basil, oregano, and red pepper.

CALORIES 80
SUGAR 4 g
(1 tsp)

DELALLO PREMIUM SAUCE, MUSHROOM

(½ cup)

If you want to skip the meat, opt for this sauce with the robust flavor of earthy mushrooms.

CALORIES 50
SUGAR 4 g
(1 tsp)

365 EVERYDAY VALUE ORGANIC FOUR CHEESE PASTA SAUCE

(½ cup)

Parmesan, Romano, provolone, and Muenster cheeses give this sauce its gutsy flavor.

CALORIES 70
SUGAR 4 g
(1 tsp)

YELLOW BARN PASTA SAUCE, ARRABBIATA

(½ cup)

This spicy sauce has only six ingredients: tomatoes, garlic, EVOO, parsley, red pepper, and salt.

CALORIES 80
SUGAR 4 g
(1 tsp)

SMART SWAP
TOMATO BISQUE

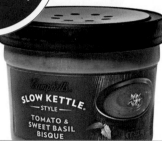

Aim for less than 250 calories and no more than five grams of added sugar per cup of canned soup.

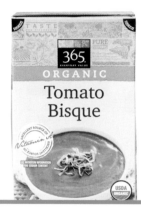

Sugar Shock
CAMPBELL'S SLOW KETTLE STYLE TOMATO & SWEET BASIL BISQUE
(1 cup)
Double the sugar if you eat the whole single-serve container as Campbell's recommends.

CALORIES 255
SUGAR 22 g (5"½ tsp)

Smart Swap
365 EVERYDAY VALUE ORGANIC TOMATO BISQUE
(1 cup)
This Whole Foods brand is a more reasonable indulgence.

CALORIES 120
SUGAR 6 g (1½ tsp)

SMART SWAPS
SOUPS

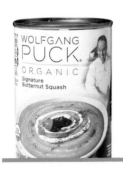 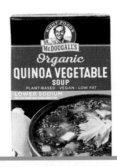 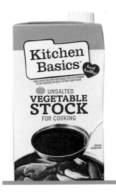 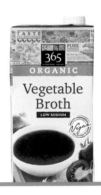

Sugar Shock → Smart Swap

WOLFGANG PUCK ORGANIC SIGNATURE BUTTERNUT SQUASH SOUP

(1 cup)

The only thing signature about this soup from a star chef are the three varieties of added sugar.

CALORIES 180

SUGAR 8 g (2 tsp)

DR. MCDOUGALL'S RIGHT FOODS ORGANIC QUINOA VEGETABLE LOWER SODIUM SOUP

(1 cup)

Quinoa adds filling protein to this chunky vegetable soup.

CALORIES 70

SUGAR 2 g (½ tsp)

Sugar Shock → Smart Swap

KITCHEN BASICS UNSALTED VEGETABLE COOKING STOCK

(1 cup)

To compensate for the lack of salt, Kitchen Basics adds sugar.

CALORIES 25

SUGAR 4 g (1 tsp)

365 EVERYDAY VALUE ORGANIC LOW SODIUM VEGETABLE BROTH

(1 cup)

If you're looking to reduce sodium in your diet, go with broths from Whole Foods, as they're all sugar-free.

CALORIES 10

SUGAR 0 g (0 tsp)

The Healthiest Soup

A can of soup is okay in a pinch, but the healthiest soup is made from scratch. Use these tricks to whip up a sugar-free soup in just minutes.

- **START WITH LOW-SODIUM CHICKEN OR VEGETABLE BROTH.** Add a can of diced tomatoes (without added sugar).
- **ADD AS MANY VEGETABLES AS POSSIBLE.** Chopped carrots, onion, celery, fennel, bell peppers, potatoes, and broccoli are good choices.
- **SEASON WITH FRESH OR DRIED HERBS.** Thyme, rosemary, parsley, dill, and/or basil are all full of flavor.
- **MAKE IT A COMPLETE MEAL WITH PROTEIN.** Add a lean protein like ready-to-eat cooked lentils, canned beans, diced tofu, or rotisserie chicken breast. Cook about 4 minutes until hot.
- **STIR IN EXTRA GREENS.** Just before serving, add a few handfuls of baby spinach or kale. Simmer about two minutes or until wilted.

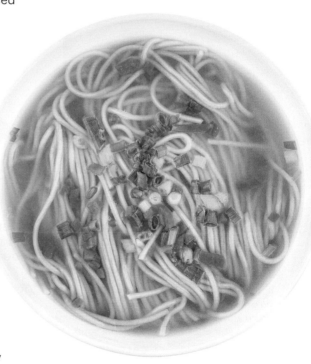

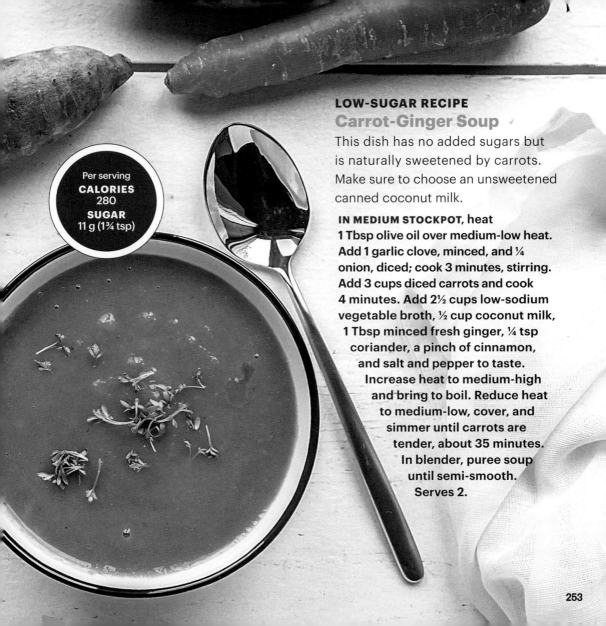

LOW-SUGAR RECIPE
Carrot-Ginger Soup

This dish has no added sugars but is naturally sweetened by carrots. Make sure to choose an unsweetened canned coconut milk.

IN MEDIUM STOCKPOT, heat 1 Tbsp olive oil over medium-low heat. Add 1 garlic clove, minced, and ¼ onion, diced; cook 3 minutes, stirring. Add 3 cups diced carrots and cook 4 minutes. Add 2½ cups low-sodium vegetable broth, ½ cup coconut milk, 1 Tbsp minced fresh ginger, ¼ tsp coriander, a pinch of cinnamon, and salt and pepper to taste. Increase heat to medium-high and bring to boil. Reduce heat to medium-low, cover, and simmer until carrots are tender, about 35 minutes. In blender, puree soup until semi-smooth. Serves 2.

Per serving
CALORIES
280
SUGAR
11 g (1¾ tsp)

253

SMART SWAP
CHILI

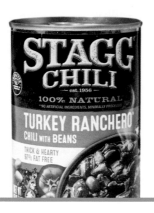 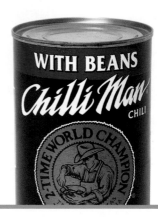

Sugar Shock → **Smart Swap**

STAGG TURKEY RANCHERO CHILI WITH BEANS

(1 cup)

Stagg says "100% Natural" on its label, but the added sugar is anything but healthy.

CALORIES 260

SUGAR 8 g (2 tsp)

CHILLI MAN LEAN BEEF CHILI WITH BEANS

(1 cup)

This version has less sugar than most major brands.

CALORIES 310

SUGAR 1 g (¼ tsp)

SMART SWAP
BAKED BEANS

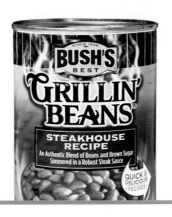 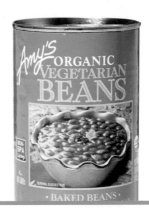

Sugar Shock	→	Smart Swap

Sugar Shock

BUSH'S BEST GRILLIN' BEANS STEAKHOUSE RECIPE

(½ cup)

Help yourself to these beans and you'll quickly blow through your daily limit of added sugar.

CALORIES 180

SUGAR 21 g (5¼ tsp)

Smart Swap

AMY'S ORGANIC VEGETARIAN BAKED BEANS

(½ cup)

If you crave baked beans, Amy's has the least added sugar of all major brands.

CALORIES 170

SUGAR 10 g (2½ tsp)

BARBEQUE SAUCES

When you're considering buying barbecue sauce, smoky flavors should come to mind, not sweet ones. But if you aren't looking at labels, a sugar bomb will sneak right by you.

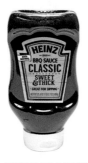

HEINZ CLASSIC ORIGINAL BBQ SAUCE
(2 Tbsp)
CALORIES 70
SUGAR 16 g
(4 tsp)

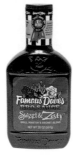

FAMOUS DAVE'S SWEET & ZESTY BBQ SAUCE
(2 Tbsp)
CALORIES 70
SUGAR 15 g
(3¾ tsp)

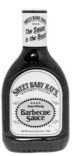

SWEET BABY RAY'S ORIGINAL BBQ SAUCE
(2 Tbsp)
CALORIES 70
SUGAR 16 g
(4 tsp)

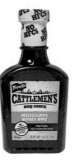

CATTLEMEN'S MISSISSIPPI HONEY BBQ SAUCE
(2 Tbsp)
CALORIES 70
SUGAR 13 g
(3¼ tsp)

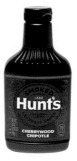

HUNT'S CHERRYWOOD CHIPOTLE BARBECUE SAUCE
(2 Tbsp)
CALORIES 70
SUGAR 13 g
(3¼ tsp)

More sugar than six Hershey's Kisses!

SMART SWAPS
BARBEQUE SAUCES

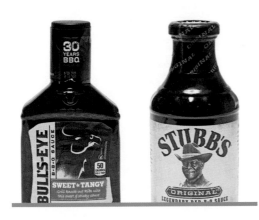
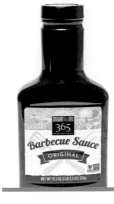
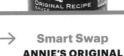

Sugar Shock →	Smart Swap	Sugar Shock →	Smart Swap
BULL'S-EYE SWEET & TANGY BARBECUE SAUCE	**STUBB'S ORIGINAL BAR-B-Q SAUCE**	**365 EVERYDAY VALUE ORGANIC BARBECUE SAUCE**	**ANNIE'S ORIGINAL BBQ SAUCE**
(2 Tbsp)	(2 Tbsp)	(2 Tbsp)	(2 Tbsp)
Another sauce with HFCS as the first ingredient.	Not only does Stubb's slash the calories and sugar in half, but it drops the HFCS for more authentic flavor.	Whole Foods BBQ sauce may be organic, but it's still too sweet.	Same organic cred—but with less than half the sugar.
CALORIES 50	**CALORIES** 25	**CALORIES** 50	**CALORIES** 35
SUGAR 11 g (2¾ tsp)	**SUGAR** 4 g (1 tsp)	**SUGAR** 11 g (2¾ tsp)	**SUGAR** 5 g (1¼ tsp)

SMART SWAP
HOISIN SAUCE

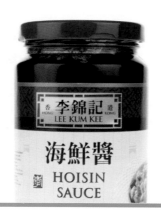
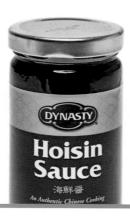

Sugar Shock
LEE KUM KEE HOISIN SAUCE

(2 Tbsp)

Buyer beware: Sugar is
the first ingredient.

CALORIES 90
SUGAR 18 g (4½ tsp)

→

Smart Swap
DYNASTY HOISIN SAUCE

(2 Tbsp)

By no means low in sugar,
Dynasty still manages to slash the
sweet stuff by more than half.

CALORIES 60
SUGAR 8 g (2 tsp)

SMART SWAP
TERIYAKI SAUCE

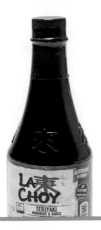

Sugar Shock
LA CHOY TERIYAKI MARINADE & SAUCE
(1 Tbsp)
Corn syrup is the primary sweetener.

CALORIES 40
SUGAR 8 g (2 tsp)

→

Smart Swap
ORGANICVILLE ISLAND TERIYAKI SAUCE & MARINADE
(1 Tbsp)
Unlike most major brands of teriyaki sauce, Organicville subs in agave nectar for typical HFCS. Bonus: Because agave is sweeter than corn syrup, you need less.

CALORIES 20
SUGAR 2 g (½ tsp)

SMART SWAP
KETCHUP

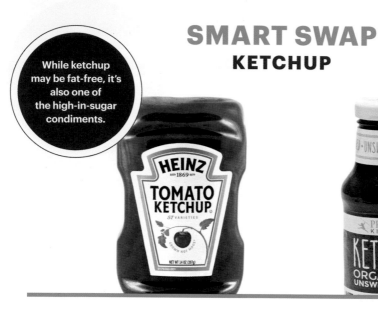

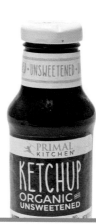

While ketchup may be fat-free, it's also one of the high-in-sugar condiments.

Sugar Shock
HEINZ TOMATO KETCHUP
(1 Tbsp)
With this much sugar, you might as well sprinkle your fries with a packet of the white stuff.

CALORIES 20
SUGAR 4 g (1 tsp)

→

Smart Swap
PRIMAL KITCHEN ORGANIC UNSWEETENED KETCHUP
(1 Tbsp)
No added sugar, just tomatoes and sweet balsamic vinegar make Primal Kitchen our pick over other sugar-free brands that contain sucralose (a.k.a. fake sugar).

CALORIES 10
SUGAR 1 g (¼ tsp)

SMART SWAP
STEAK SAUCE

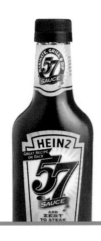
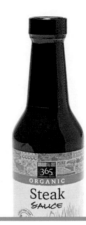

Sugar Shock

HEINZ 57 SAUCE

(1 Tbsp)

Unfortunately, Heinz makes
its sauce with HFCS too.

CALORIES 20
SUGAR 4 g (1 tsp)

→

Smart Swap

**365 EVERYDAY VALUE ORGANIC
STEAK SAUCE**

(1 Tbsp)

Whole Foods skips the
HFCS and slashes the sweet
so you can feel better
about saucing your steak.

CALORIES 10
SUGAR 1 g (¼ tsp)

SMART SWAPS
SNACKS

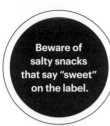

Beware of salty snacks that say "sweet" on the label.

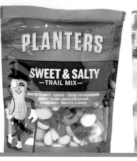

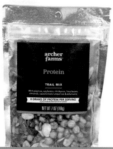

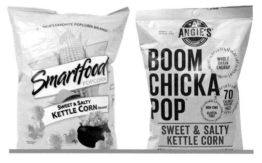

Sugar Shock →

PLANTERS SWEET & SALTY TRAIL MIX

(3 Tbsp)

M&M'S and yogurt-coated raisins make this trail mix a sugar bomb.

CALORIES 150

SUGAR 11 g (2¾ tsp)

Smart Swap

ARCHER FARMS PROTEIN TRAIL MIX

(¼ cup)

It's packed with protein thanks to dried soybeans, chickpeas, and fava beans. The only sweet in Target's brand is from dried cranberries.

CALORIES 140

SUGAR 2 g (½ tsp)

Sugar Shock →

SMARTFOOD SWEET & SALTY KETTLE CORN FLAVORED POPCORN

(1¼ cups)

This kettle corn may be labeled "smart" but it's still too sweet.

CALORIES 140

SUGAR 12 g (3 tsp)

Smart Swap

ANGIE'S BOOM CHICKA POP SWEET & SALTY KETTLE CORN

(3¼ cups)

If you want to enjoy kettle corn, this "light" version is a much better choice.

CALORIES 120

SUGAR 5 g (1¼ tsp)

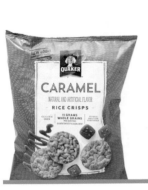
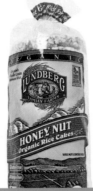
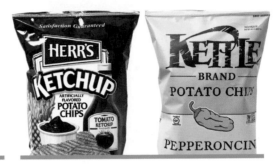

Sugar Shock →
QUAKER RICE CAKES, CARAMEL CORN

(1 cake/13 g)

Added sugars include fructose and maltodextrin.

CALORIES 50
SUGAR 3 g (¾ tsp)

Smart Swap
LUNDBERG FAMILY FARMS HONEY NUT ORGANIC RICE CAKES

(1 cake/21 g)

Lundberg uses whole-grain brown rice (versus processed white rice) and half the sweeteners for a healthier treat.

CALORIES 80
SUGAR 2 g (½ tsp)

Sugar Shock →
HERR'S POTATO CHIPS, KETCHUP

(13 chips/1 oz)

Best to take a pass on this sugary attempt to mimic the flavor of ketchup and fries.

CALORIES 150
SUGAR 3 g (¾ tsp)

Smart Swap
KETTLE POTATO CHIPS, PEPPERONCINI

(13 chips/1 oz)

The better choice: tangy vinegar chips seasoned with two types of pepper.

CALORIES 140
SUGAR 0 g (0 tsp)

SMART SWAP
BEEF JERKY

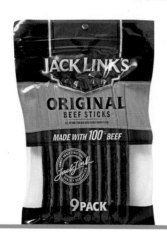 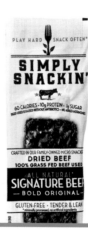

Sugar Shock

**JACK'S LINKS ORIGINAL
BEEF STICKS**

(1 oz)

Like other major brands of
beef jerky, America's top seller
has plenty of added sugar.

CALORIES 80

SUGAR 6 g (1½ tsp)

→

Smart Swap

**SIMPLY SNACKIN' SIGNATURE
BEEF, BOLD ORIGINAL**

(1 oz)

Dried beef from Simply Snackin'
has the same beefy taste but only
a fraction of the added sugar.

CALORIES 60

SUGAR 1 g (¼ tsp)

SMART SWAPS
CHIPS & CRACKERS

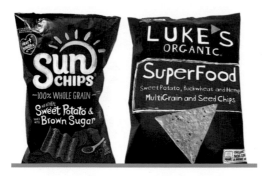

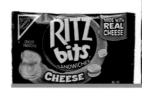

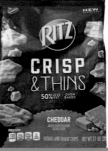

Sugar Shock →

SUNCHIPS SWEET POTATO & BROWN SUGAR WHOLE GRAIN SNACKS

(14 chips/28 g)

"Whole-grain snacks" may sound better than potato chips, but not when they're sweetened with brown sugar.

CALORIES 140

SUGAR 3 g (¾ tsp)

Smart Swap

LUKE'S ORGANIC SUPERFOOD SWEET POTATO, HEMP & BUCKWHEAT MULTIGRAIN & SEED CHIPS

(12 chips/1 oz)

Same sweet potato chips minus the added sugar (plus quinoa to boost the protein).

CALORIES 140

SUGAR 0 g (0 tsp)

Sugar Shock →

RITZ BITS SANDWICHES, CHEESE

(13 sandwiches/31 g)

Might want to skip these sweet cracker snacks with processed cheese filling.

CALORIES 160

SUGAR 4 g (1 tsp)

Smart Swap

RITZ CRISP & THINS, CHEDDAR

(21 chips/30 g)

These cheesy chips from Ritz are half as sweet.

CALORIES 130

SUGAR 2 g (½ tsp)

SMART SWAPS
CRACKERS

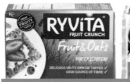 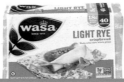

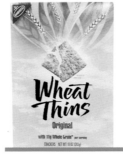 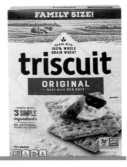

Sugar Shock → **Smart Swap**

RYVITA FRUIT & OATS RYE CRISPBREAD

(2 slices/30 g)

This crispbread with currants and honey may taste great with cheese, but it's best to take a pass if you're watching your sugar intake.

CALORIES 100

SUGAR 6 g (1½ tsp)

WASA LIGHT RYE CRISPBREAD

(2 slices/18 g)

Wasa delivers just as much fiber but with far fewer calories and no added sweeteners.

CALORIES 40

SUGAR 0 g (0 tsp)

Sugar Shock → **Smart Swap**

WHEAT THINS ORIGINAL WHOLE GRAIN CRACKERS

(16 crackers/31 g)

Three types of added sugars are not what you need in a cracker.

CALORIES 140

SUGAR 5 g (1¼ tsp)

TRISCUIT ORIGINAL WHOLE GRAIN WHEAT CRACKERS

(6 crackers/28 g)

You'll find three grams of filling fiber in every serving.

CALORIES 120

SUGAR 0 g (0 tsp)

FIVE SUGAR-FREE
CRACKERS

Check out these crispbreads and crackers without a trace of added sweet.

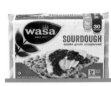
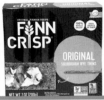
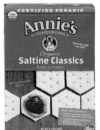
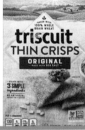
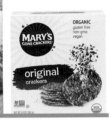

WASA WHOLE GRAIN CRISPBREAD, SOURDOUGH

(1 slice/12 g)

Top a hearty crispbread with cottage cheese and fresh berries for the perfect snack.

CALORIES 30

SUGAR 0 g

(0 tsp)

FINN CRISP ORIGINAL SOURDOUGH RYE THINS

(1 slice/7 g)

With a rich rye taste and extra-crunchy texture, these crispbreads are excellent topped with smoked salmon or smoked cheese.

CALORIES 20

SUGAR 0 g

(0 tsp)

ANNIE'S ORGANIC SALTINE CLASSICS

(7 crackers/15 g)

Spread these classic crackers with your favorite nut butter.

CALORIES 70

SUGAR 0 g

(0 tsp)

TRISCUIT THIN CRISPS CRACKERS, ORIGINAL

(15 crackers/30 g)

Whole-grain wheat, canola oil, and sea salt are the only ingredients you'll find on the front of the box.

CALORIES 130

SUGAR 0 g

(0 tsp)

MARY'S GONE CRACKERS, ORIGINAL CRACKERS

(13 crackers/30 g)

Brown rice, quinoa, flaxseeds, and sesame seeds make these crackers extra crunchy.

CALORIES 140

SUGAR 0 g

(0 tsp)

HEARST
HOME

Cover design by Trevor Richardson
Book design by Sabrina Contratti

Library of Congress Cataloging-in-Publication Data Available on Request

10 9 8 7 6 5 4 3 2 1

Published by Hearst Home, an imprint of Hearst Books/Hearst Magazine Media, Inc.

Hearst Magazine Media, Inc.
300 West 57th Street
New York, NY 10019

Hearst Home, the Hearst Home logo, and Hearst Books are registered trademarks of Hearst Magazine Media, Inc.

For information about custom editions, special sales, premium and corporate purchases, please go to hearst.com/magazines/hearst-books

Printed in China
ISBN 978-1-950785-00-1